About the Book

*r*eclaiming *Your Life After Diagnosis* is packed with all of the most important information and resources to get you or someone you love through the challenging journey of a cancer diagnosis, treatment, and beyond. Backed by the Cancer Support Community (www.cancersupportcommunity.org), one of the largest, most respected cancer organizations in the world, this one book tells you everything you need to know to address your physical, emotional, financial, social, and practical needs.

Complete with Patient Action Plans detailing actions you can take each step of the way, *Reclaiming Your Life After Diagnosis* allows you to empower yourself to become actively involved in your treatment and long-term well-being. Find out how to

- put a strong support and resource team in place to buffer against the challenges of diagnosis, treatment, and survivorship;
- educate yourself on different treatments and identify, with the help of your doctor, what treatment plan is right for you;
- develop practical, more effective ways to manage side effects;
- deal with complex emotional issues ranging from the shock of initial diagnosis to creating a living legacy and a meaning-filled life.

With powerful stories from real patients and survivors, evidence-based research, and the best treatment and support information available, *Reclaiming Your Life After Diagnosis* will help you develop the strength you need to stay focused on healing—to live longer and better.

reclaiming
your life
after
diagnosis

The Cancer Support
Community Handbook

CANCER SUPPORT COMMUNITY

Kim Thiboldeaux

President and CEO

AND **Mitch Golant, PhD**
Senior Vice President of Research and Training

BENBELLA BOOKS, INC.
D A L L A S ,   T E X A S

This publication is designed to provide accurate and authoritative information in regard to the subject matter covered. It is sold with the understanding that the publisher is not engaged in rendering medical, legal, or other professional services. If medical advice or other professional assistance is required, the services of a competent professional person should be sought.
—Adapted from a Declaration of Principles jointly adopted by a committee of the American Bar Association and a Committee of Publishers and Associations

BENBELLA

BenBella Books, Inc.
10300 N. Central Expy, Suite 400
Dallas, TX 75231
www.benbellabooks.com
Send feedback to feedback@benbellabooks.com

Printed in the United States of America
10 9 8 7 6 5 4 3 2 1

Library of Congress Cataloging-in-Publication Data

Thiboldeaux, Kim.

Reclaiming Your Life After Diagnosis: The Cancer Support Community Handbook / by Kim Thiboldeaux, and Mitch Golant.
p. cm.
ISBN 978-1-936661-76-3
   1. Cancer—Popular works. 2. Cancer—Psychological aspects. I. Golant, Mitch. II. Title.

RC263.T45 2007
616.99'4—dc22
2007006819

Editing by Dorianne R. Perrucci
Copyediting by Laura Kidder
Proofreading by Cape Cod Compositors and Brittany Dowdle
Cover design by Allison Bard
Photo of Kim Thiboldeaux by Connie Reider
Photo of Mitch Golant by Lee Moskow
Text design and composition by John Reinhardt Book Design
Printed by Bang Printing

This book is dedicated to the memory of our dear friends and late founders of The Wellness Community, Dr. Harold Benjamin and his wife Harriet Benjamin, and to the vision of the founder of Gilda's Club, Joanna Bull, MA, MFCC. We are so pleased that these two legacy organizations, The Wellness Community and Gilda's Club Worldwide, have joined forces to become the Cancer Support Community.

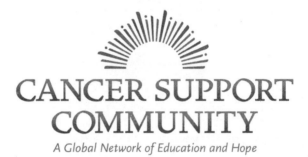

CANCER SUPPORT COMMUNITY
A Global Network of Education and Hope

Contents

Part Four: Moving from Patient to Survivor

Foreword

tHE NEWS ABOUT CANCER is better than ever. Even though more people are being diagnosed, fewer people are dying from the disease, and people are living longer and better with cancer. They're also learning how to live well with, through, and beyond it.

In the last twenty-five years, there have been dramatic advances in the diagnosis and treatment of cancer. These advances across most cancers have resulted in improved outcomes, leading to larger numbers than ever before of disease-free, long-term survivors, as well as prolonged survival for those who have developed *metastatic* disease.

But as the number of those living with cancer rises, so does the burden on the health care system. As a result, patients are finding themselves in the position of having to take control of their own care plans. In essence, they have become empowered health care consumers. In a *New York Times*/CBS News poll of 1,111 adults in February 2005, 44 percent of patients who received a diagnosis sought more information about treatment options from sources who were not their physicians— including the Internet, friends, relatives, and even other doctors. Slightly more than half of surveyed patients who received a diagnosis were given multiple treatment options—and one-third made the decision on their own. Those between 45 and 64 years old were most likely to take their medical care into their own hands by making informed, educated decisions about their treatments.

Patients need to work to overcome the three most common stressors from cancer: loss of hope, loss of control, and a sense of isolation. They must become educated and empowered. More than ever, today's cancer patient is captain of his or her own treatment team.

Still, unless cancer patients have effective support and resource teams in place to buffer against the trauma of the diagnosis and treatment, as well as to help navigate the many choices they have in every aspect of this life-transforming disease, they and their families will struggle daily with daunting decisions that most of us hope we will never have to make. In many ways, it takes a village—a cancer support community—to help guide the patient through the labyrinth of choices in dealing with issues ranging from dealing with the shock of initial diagnosis to creating a living legacy and a meaningful life.

Through powerful, first-person testimonies from members of the Cancer Support Community, as well as a plethora of the best tips, evidence-based research, treatment, and support information currently available, *Reclaiming Your Life After Diagnosis: The Cancer Support Community Handbook*, will help you, the cancer patient, feel empowered, positive, and focused on healing. You'll learn how to live well with your disease—no matter what the road ahead may bring.

Wherever you are in the continuum of the cancer experience (newly diagnosed, in active treatment, in post-treatment, or a long-term survivor), this book has something to offer you.

— *Mehmet Oz, MD*, Professor and Vice Chair,
  NY Presbyterian/Columbia

The Cancer Support Community:

A Bold New Vision in Cancer Care

When you have cancer, you don't focus on what's happened. Rather you look forward to what is to come and what will be—that's called survival.

MADELINE,
advanced breast cancer survivor

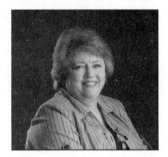

I N THE UNITED STATES there are currently 12 million cancer survivors who need support and hope to continue to live well. Unfortunately, those numbers are projected to increase significantly as more people are diagnosed with cancer every year. In 2012, approximately 1.6 million more people will be diagnosed—and that number is expected to increase dramatically as 77 million Baby Boomers age.

At the Cancer Support Community (CSC), we are committed to providing the comprehensive care this growing population needs. CSC formed in 2009, when The Wellness Community and Gilda's Club Worldwide, two of the foremost cancer-support organizations in the United States, joined forces. We base the foundation of our work on the pivotal report issued in 2007 by the Institute of Medicine (IOM) in Washington, D.C. *Cancer Care for the Whole Patient: Meeting Psychosocial Health Needs,* which states that, "Today, it is not possible to deliver good-quality cancer care without addressing patients' psychosocial health needs." This means that comprehensive cancer care must address the social, emotional, spiritual, and financial impact of a diagnosis. In addition, we are beginning to see an important shift in medical care, known as "patient-centered" care, that recognizes that the patient and his or her family must be at the center of care and actively involved in making key decisions and setting medical and life priorities. The Cancer Support Community is taking the lead in ensuring that people with cancer receive the best possible care, so that *all* of their needs are met, as described in this landmark IOM report. This book will help guide the growing number of cancer patients—and survivors, whose numbers have quadrupled since 1970—on how to do just that.

CSC's programs are for people of all ages with any type or stage of cancer. Online and onsite CSC services such as professionally led support groups, educational workshops, nutrition and exercise programs, and stress-reduction classes empower people affected by cancer to learn vital skills that enable them to regain control, reduce isolation, and restore hope—regardless of the stage of their disease.

With more than forty-five years of history, CSC is empowering people affected by cancer to live better lives in the face of cancer; addressing individual needs and creating strong links to a community of support and hope. Currently there are fifty CSC affiliate locations around the United States; more than one hundred satellite locations; centers abroad in Israel, Japan, and Canada, ten affiliates in development; and a wide range of resources, support programs, and networking opportunities online at www.cancersupportcommunity.org. As a leader in the field, we also partner with a wide variety of organizations that include our own community-based affiliates, hospitals, community oncology practices, and research institutions and other nonprofit organizations to ensure that patients and families are getting the care, support, and resources they need to manage a cancer diagnosis.

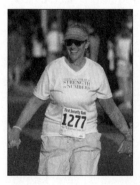

The cancer journey is difficult. That's why it's best to take it with the support of friends and loved ones. The Cancer Support Community provided me and my caregivers with additional strength by hosting a support group of wonderful women (Bosom Buddies) and many other helpful programs. After five years of cancer survivorship, I remain very active with this community, which has given so much to me. Now I can try to give a little back to others facing this journey.

MARION CHERRY,
community member, Cancer Support Community, Montana

About This Book

There are plenty of books available about cancer. Some are clinical, while others are personal journeys from survivors offering advice on everything from choosing the right doctor to alternative care. Like many other people with cancer, you might be looking for one book that tells you just about everything you need to know—in a positive, honest, and easy-to-understand manner. If so, you will most definitely benefit from the broad scope of detail in this book. *Reclaiming Your Life After Diagnosis: The Cancer Support Community Handbook* contains facts about cancer, treatment options, and side-effect management, without forgetting that you are a human being faced with major life issues. More than anything else, you need to hear from others who have *really* been there, done that, and are inspired to tell about it. Like them, you'll want to be an active participant in your own treatment—to grow from this experience and to regain your sense of control and hope.

Guidance, Support, and Powerful Action Plans

Broken into four sections that span the cancer continuum from diagnosis through a sometimes unpredictable future, *Reclaiming Your Life After Diagnosis* is the first book to cover everything you and your family need to know about being active participants in your own long-term plan for well-being. With so many cancer patients becoming survivors, living longer and better has become an increasingly important point of focus for the Cancer Support Community and its team of experts. At the end of each chapter, you'll find a *Patient Action Plan* with specific steps you can take now. These will help you put the main concepts expressed in each chapter to practical and immediate use.

With accurate information and compassionate understanding, this book addresses the physical, emotional, social, and practical needs of today's cancer patient, caregiver, and survivor—preparing you for wellness that can follow you throughout the rest of your life.

Join us at a CSC affiliate near you—or anytime online at www.cancersupportcommunity.org. We're here for you!

> *I came through the red doors and it was like a breath of fresh air. They all treated me like they had known me for years.*
>
> COMMUNITY MEMBER,
> *Gilda's Club, Desert Cities*

Part One

Becoming Empowered

Chapter 1

Understanding Cancer

Cancer changes many of the day-to-day aspects of living, but the pursuit of happiness can go on during the fight for recovery if you want it to.

HAROLD BENJAMIN,
founder, The Wellness Community
(now the Cancer Support Community)

THE NATIONAL CANCER ACT of 1971 declared a "War on Cancer" that started a significant crusade against a deadly disease. Since then, many strides have been made to improve early detection and develop safer and more effective treatments. In fact, the number of cancer survivors in the United States has quadrupled since 1970. Some cancers have had dramatic increases in cure rates, including Hodgkin's disease; specific blood, testicular, and thyroid cancers; and some childhood cancers. Yet, as our population ages, more and more people will be diagnosed with cancer. In 2012, it is estimated that 1.6 million Americans will be diagnosed. That translates to one in *every* two men and one in *every* three women who will be diagnosed with cancer in their lifetime. According to the National Cancer Institute (NCI), cancer has replaced heart disease as the leading cause of U.S. deaths for people under the age of 85.

Fortunately, thanks to a greater awareness of the ways that cancer can impact a person's entire life, treatment is becoming more comprehensive. In addition to medical advances, increased attention is now being paid to social and emotional well-being, with a focus on quality of life after diagnosis. The Cancer Support Community (CSC) has dedicated many years to addressing the issues of quality of life and the fight for recovery, as an integral part of the medical care for people affected by cancer.

What Is Cancer?

The term "cancer" is a generic name that applies to more than one hundred diseases that share similar characteristics. Cancer occurs when

- an abnormal cell appears in the body;
- the cell continues to divide and subdivide after it should have stopped;
- the new cells eventually form a clump, called a tumor, which, if unchecked, will grow large enough to interfere with the delivery of nutrients and oxygen to nearby organs.

Cancer cells can survive in parts of the body other than where they originated.

This is called *metastasis*.

Our bodies consist of a collection of cells that perform specific functions. Each is linked to the others, operating in a highly regulated manner. In a normal cycle, a cell is born, matures, performs its designated function, and then "dies." At this point, it must be replaced by a new cell. This is accomplished when a nearby cell divides in half, and then those two divide, and so on, until the exact number of required new cells is reached. Under normal circumstances, the birth and death of a cell is an exquisitely precise process.

Problems arise when, for reasons still unknown, a normal cell divides to replace other cells and gives birth to an abnormal cell. This abnormal cell does not stop dividing when it is supposed to and refuses to die on schedule. Such cells, if unchecked, divide and subdivide endlessly and eventually join together to form a tumor. As the tumor becomes larger, it impedes the functioning of nearby organs by intruding on their space and interfering with their supply of oxygen and nutrients. Eventually, unless the growth is stopped, or the tumor is removed, the healthy organs are destroyed.

There are two types of abnormal cells. The first can survive only at its place of origin and forms a tumor where it originates. This is called a benign tumor, which can often be surgically removed, thereby ending the problem. The other type of abnormal cell, called a malignant cell, is more dangerous, because it does not stop dividing when it is supposed to and can thrive any place in the body. This ability to travel and survive in other parts of the body is called metastasis. Cancer cells can form a tumor at the primary site (the breast, colon, or lung), as well as in other parts of the body where the tumor has metastasized.

For cancer to be treated successfully, not only must the original tumor be identified and controlled, but the spread of disease, or metastasis, must also be stopped.

A leading contemporary theory states that abnormal cells may commonly proliferate in our bodies as a normal course of health. The reason that these proliferating cells do not become cancerous may be that our immune systems are strong enough to destroy

> *In 2010, the National Institutes of Health estimated that the overall cost of cancer was $263.8 billion—and that cost is rising.*

the cancer cells as they appear. Video has actually shown cancer cells being attacked and destroyed by immune system cells, as if in battle. It's an inspiring sight. Some cancer patients use that image to visualize their bodies responding in a proactive manner.

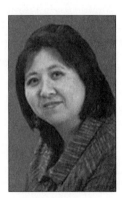

> *I remember when my Mom was first diagnosed with cancer. This was a totally foreign experience. I didn't know who to turn to or what to do about it. By coming to The Wellness Community, I found a connection with people—something I really needed. I knew that I could find other resources that would help us too.*
>
> TILDA,
> *long-distance caregiver*

The Immune System: Our First Line of Defense

The immune system is intricately designed to protect the body from disease. It can also defend against "foreigners" that invade through a break in the skin, via food or other ingested matter, in the air we breathe, or through the rays to which we are exposed. For cancer to take hold, the malignant cell appears when the immune system is too weak to rid the body of it, or it does not recognize the cancer cell to be a problem worth fighting. This view of cancer is generally known as the immune surveillance theory.

Myths about Cancer

Despite the fact that cancer has been a leading cause of death for decades, not everything you hear about it is true. Take a closer look at the truths behind some popular misconceptions.

- **Myth: Cancer is a death sentence.**
  Today there are 12 million cancer survivors—in 1970 there were 3 million. The fact is, with better screening and treatment, more people are living with cancer—and beyond —than ever before.

- **Myth: You are powerless against cancer.**
  There are actions, behaviors, and attitudes that you, your physician, and your health care team can use that will not only improve your quality of life, but also might enhance the possibility of recovery.

- **Myth: Surgery causes cancer to grow and spread.**
  Surgery is often an important part of a successful treatment plan for cancer. Surgery does not affect the spread of cancer.

- **Myth: Disfiguring surgery is always part of cancer treatment.**
  Some people with cancer need surgery, and some people do not. If you need surgery, you should know that reconstructive and plastic surgery is often used to avoid and correct disfiguring effects.

- **Myth: Terrible pain that cannot be relieved is part of cancer or its treatment.**
  Some people do have pain with their cancer or treatment; other people do not. Most pain is treatable and can be relieved with modern pain-relief medicine and other treatments.

- **Myth: Chemotherapy will make you sick each time you get it.**
  There are many medications and other treatments that are now given to help control the side effects of *chemotherapy*. They help you feel and stay well during and after your chemotherapy treatment.

- **Myth: Radiation treatment burns off your skin.**
  There are many skin-care treatments and other medications that can be used to protect your skin in preparation and during radiation.
- **Myth: Chemotherapy will always make your hair fall out.**
  Only some chemotherapy makes you lose your hair and, even then, only temporarily. It grows back a few months after treatment, but it may look somewhat different.
- **Myth: Having cancer and getting treatments means that you will be in the hospital all of the time.**
  Most cancer treatment is provided on an outpatient basis. Ask your doctor and nurse what you can expect.

Gain Knowledge about Cancer Research Today

By 2020, the Healthy People goals established by the U.S. government have set the bar to reduce the number of new cancer cases, as well as the illness, disability, and death caused by cancer. In response, new categories of drugs are being developed to treat the disease, and scientists are exploring new mechanisms to better understand how the cancer cell functions at the most basic genetic level.

While some cancers can be cured, others may never entirely disappear and may require ongoing treatment to be controlled. As a result, many patients are living longer after a cancer diagnosis and often must learn how to achieve and maintain a better quality of life. In fact, for some, cancer can become a chronic illness to be managed and controlled over the course of many years until new treatments are discovered.

The number of people affected by cancer is increasing, as a result of improved early detection and better cancer treatments. Today, there are over 12 million cancer survivors alive in the United States, compared to only 3 million in 1970.

For the last several decades, common treatments have included surgery, radiation, and chemotherapy. While these are focused on destroying the tumor cells, they can damage normal cells as well. The newest category of cancer treatments are targeted therapies. These act in specialized ways to destroy or interfere with tumor cell growth, often not affecting normal cells. As a result, targeted treatment harms only cancer cells, causing fewer of the traditional treatment side effects, such as hair loss and nausea. The newer treatments can also be combined with older therapies to enhance their effectiveness. You will find more information about how targeted therapies work, including details about cell growth and death, hormones, the immune system, and aspects of genes later in this book.

Patient Action Plan

- **Research your cancer.**
  Gain as much knowledge as you can, as soon as you discover you have cancer. Know that knowledge is power.
- **Learn from others.**
  Seek out cancer support groups or organizations that can connect you with someone who's been there. You are not alone.
- **It's more than okay to ask questions.**
  Learn to become comfortable with asking your doctors any question that you have about cancer, support, and recovery.
- **Understand that cancer research is ongoing, and new treatments are always on the horizon.**
  Ask about clinical trials or innovations.

Chapter 2

Regaining Your Balance After Diagnosis

One sleet-gray March day, the color of dying ashes, the sky the color of Mark Twain's mustache, (my doctor) announced: "You have cancer." My face turned gray....I heard distinctly, "You are going to die."

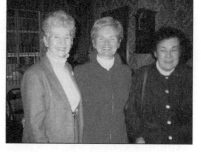

EILEEN O'DONNELL,
self-described "cancer-thriver" and community member,
Cancer Support Community, Greater Lehigh Valley

F YOU'VE JUST BEEN DIAGNOSED with cancer, chances are you're in a state of shock. Often, the mere mention of the word causes alarm. You might panic.

Depending on how much you know about cancer, or through experiences you've had with others, your emotions will be raw. It's natural to expect your first reactions to be shock, grief, and resistance to the changes occurring in your life. At the very least, the news is sobering. However, it's important to remember that we live in a time when more cancers are being treated successfully. Nevertheless, common problems around gathering information, feelings of anxiety, financial worries, and difficulties with practical logistics (for example, getting to and from treatments or finding a babysitter) can cause disabling distress, if not depression.

What can you do to help yourself? First, take a deep breath. Realize that you are the same person you were just a moment before you learned that you were ill. Second—and this isn't meant to seem contradictory—realize that the one thing you can expect is that cancer will change your life. Some things might actually be better than before; paradoxically, cancer can bring certain gifts. Conversely, your circumstances may change in ways you consider more negative. Either way, the sooner you can adjust to the fact that your life has changed, the sooner you can participate more fully in managing your illness.

There are practical steps you can take to help you regain a sense of control over your circumstances. There are ways to regain your emotional balance. You can still be the person in the driver's seat of your life. You can control your response to the illness. You can find positives throughout your journey with this disease called cancer.

You can control your response to the illness. You can find positives throughout your journey with this disease called cancer.

And what a journey it will be! One minute you were living your life, seemingly on your own terms. In an instant, all of that changed. But you're not alone. You're actually the nucleus of a brand-new team that is devoted to taking the best possible care of you. True, you didn't choose this path, but it will nevertheless be less challenging with the love and support of your family and friends, the new friends you'll meet along the way, other patients, and a host of medical professionals who might become part of an "unofficial" extended family.

What a Cancer Diagnosis Means...and Doesn't Mean

In the last several decades, there have been dramatic advances in the diagnosis and treatment of most cancers. These developments have resulted in improved outcomes, leading to larger numbers of disease-free, long-term survivors, as well as prolonged survival for those developing metastatic diseases. The National Cancer Institute (NCI) estimates that approximately 14 percent of the 12 million cancer survivors alive today were diagnosed more than twenty years ago. Cancer is often not a death sentence, but something people must learn to live with for many years to come.

Those diagnosed today benefit from the medical profession's increased awareness of the psychological impact of cancer. Research has shown that, in general, 25–30 percent of newly diagnosed and recurrent patients experience high levels of emotional distress. While some individuals might require psychiatric counseling to help them deal with substantial distress, most everyone affected by cancer would benefit from some level of social, emotional, and practical support.

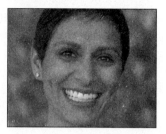

When you hear the words, "You have breast cancer," it's easy to feel like you need to make decisions within days of your diagnosis. But in most cases you have time to meet with different physicians to learn about your surgery and treatment...The Cancer Support Community taught me the importance of taking a proactive role in my decision-making, and I encourage all women to do the same.

SHARISTA,
breast cancer survivor

Acknowledge the Change Cancer Has Brought to Your Life

A generation ago, cancer was often a dark secret that we kept to ourselves and our closest family members; indeed, some people didn't even tell their families that they were sick. Conversely, some family members kept the truth from their ill loved one. Fortunately, times have changed.

Today, much can be done to counteract such isolation and distress. In fact, throughout this book, you'll find many suggested coping skills that can help you. One key is to acknowledge your diagnosis. Yell if you need to. Cry. Laugh. Share your anger,

It's not a sign of weakness to say to yourself and others that you have cancer and that you wish you didn't, but that it's simply an ongoing "part of" your life.

dismay, fear, and other emotions with caring family and friends. Find some way to acknowledge that your life has changed...and that you wish it hadn't. That one action will help dispel some of the stress you're feeling.

Some people with cancer actually create an irreverent nickname for the illness, or they refer to events in their life as "BC" (Before Cancer) or "AC" (After Cancer). They do this to incorporate the illness as part of their lives—because it's just "part of" their lives. The secret to a healthy mindset is contained in those two little words: "part of."

Failing to acknowledge the changes in your life post-diagnosis can allow the illness to loom so large, it seems insurmountable. Acknowledging its presence doesn't mean you are granting it permission to take over your life. Stay in the driver's seat by saying, "I see you. I'm dealing with you, but you don't get to become my entire life. I'm still going to be the boss."

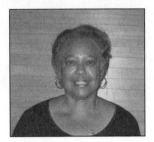

I joined The Wellness Community (now the Cancer Support Community) after my first surgery at City of Hope. I became aware of the devastating effects cancer has on so many others. As we shared stories and experiences, I learned so much about the health care system, doctors, nurses, and hospitals. I not only became better informed, I also learned how to ask the right questions.

Diane Turner,
community member, Cancer Support Community, Pasadena

Become Informed

One of the most important tools for reducing emotional stress, and becoming proactive in your care, is information. You and your family need reliable, comprehensive, and current information to help you identify the best options for treatment; to manage the disease better over time; and to feel confident that you're receiving the best care available. If it's too difficult for you to educate yourself, ask a trusted friend or family member to gather information and distill it for you.

Fortunately, people today have access to much more information about their disease and its treatment than patients did a generation ago. Obtaining, assessing, and processing that wealth of information is important since it gives you the opportunity to be a savvy consumer. It will also help you form a partnership with your medical team, rather than simply becoming a passive "body" receiving treatment.

However, bear in mind that the amount of information available is overwhelming in its content and complexity. That's why it's important to have a team helping you. Is one family member able to negotiate the maze of insurance forms on your behalf? Is a good friend a calming influence on you when you're visiting your doctor? Ask that trusted ally to accompany you and take notes while you talk with and listen to your physician, and let others help as they can. This leaves you free to concentrate fully on what's being said. You don't need to worry about forgetting the details of the conversation. Indeed, your trusted ally might be much better at gathering the best information—and less prone to the ups and downs you and close family members might be experiencing.

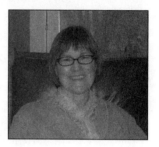

As a member of Gilda's Club, Metro Detroit, I have been empowered to live with cancer. Thirteen-and-a-half years ago, I began with a wellness group, then moved on to take yoga, nutrition, and meditation classes. I attended lectures by leading cancer experts, who gave me knowledge to make good health choices, and received social support from other members who became—and still are—a major source of strength and support. I now have more confidence to face the everyday challenges of living with cancer.

JEANNE DENEWETH,
community member, Gilda's Club, Metro Detroit

Get Organized

The sheer volume of information available about your illness can be perplexing. Sometimes it's rather technical, even when it's supposed to be user-friendly. Sometimes one source will contradict another, and you might wonder which one is "right" or more reliable. You'll also find that the information base grows exponentially. Every time you think you understand the basics of your disease, a new treatment or article comes to light and takes you down another road, or someone innocently and unknowingly shares inaccurate information. It can all be quite bewildering.

For these reasons, it becomes important to prepare for upcoming doctors' visits and for life in between. Before a doctor's visit, it is wise to prepare your list of questions and to have your trusted ally join you to keep track of all of the information. Additionally, create a file or note-book to organize data so you can refer back to it when needed. This might include separate files for: "Practical Information" (directions to the treatment center or the appropriate parking deck), "Side Effects" (if you're undergoing new treatment), "Prescriptions" (which could be a list of medications and doses you're taking), "Clinical Trials" (for research on promising innovative treatments), and so on.

Asking for specific help from your spouse or trusted ally might seem difficult at first, but this can become a special way to connect with others. For example, someone could become the "go-to" person to provide updates to friends and associates about your condition, at least at times when you're too busy or tired to deal with these conversations. Your savvy teenager could help you set up an online "social network" that would reach people near or far who wish to stay in touch. Several useful Web sites like www.mylifeline.org, www.carepages.com, and www.caringbridge .org can keep you organized and connected. These sites include calendar functions to help you track appointments and obtain help when you need it for rides to the hospital, shopping, meals, babysitting, or other tasks that suddenly seem impossible. Loved ones often want to help, but don't know how. Web sites like the ones mentioned above are excellent ways to stay organized and help you manage your schedule. If you don't have such resources among your friends and family, often someone on your medical team, such as a medical social worker, can refer you to groups that provide hands-on support for people in your situation.

Fight Depression

The emotional and social impact of cancer and its physical symptoms can lead to depression and anxiety. These stressors can influence your ability to cope with and manage the many demands that are part of the cancer experience and getting proper treatment.

Distress or even hopelessness can have many different dimensions. It's not easily described as one single emotional or physical reaction, but can range from normal feelings of vulnerability to sadness and fear to more disabling problems, such as depression, anxiety, panic, social isolation, and an existential or spiritual crisis.

A recent analysis of 31 studies found a 25 percent higher mortality rate for patients with cancer who also experienced depressive symptoms and a 39 percent higher mortality rate for those with major depression.

Does treating depression prolong survival? This question still remains unanswered. On the other hand, treating depression is critical for improving your quality of life and ability to cope with your disease. In a recent study, women with breast cancer who were diagnosed and treated for depression in the first year after joining a support group actually did live longer and reported a decrease in sadness, isolation, and depression. The important message of this research is that early detection and the treatment of depression can predict survival many years later. This study and others demonstrate the need for support services for people with cancer. The study also underscores the importance of identifying depression and other emotional concerns before they impact your life.

Stigma has been associated with cancer and depression for centuries. It might be a major barrier to your ability to ask for help, but there's good news: Depression can be assessed and treated according to clinical practice guidelines. Your emotional well-being is entirely manageable with proper screening, support, and treatment. A key ingredient to appropriate management, of course, is for you to be candid in describing your feelings with your medical team.

Just as scientists are working to discover how to detect cancer earlier, psychosocial oncology professionals would like to identify emotional distress or other social and emotional concerns earlier for people with cancer. Everyone can get the support they need to participate actively in treatment and maintain a good quality of life—throughout cancer and beyond.

You do not realize it immediately, but once you're diagnosed with cancer, you are changed. From that moment forward, you'll always be one of two things: either a cancer patient or a cancer survivor. But in either case, "cancer" is one-half of your title. I am not pleased I got cancer; however, as a result of the challenge, I'm more focused and cognizant of everything in my life that is of value.

DREW VAN DOPP,
community member, Cancer Support Community, Delmarva

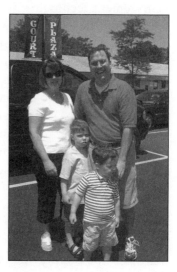

Are You Feeling Hopeless?

If you're not sure, ask someone close to you to answer a few questions.

- Have I been using negative words that indicate a feeling of doom?
- Have I been acting as if there's no reason for hope?
- Do I appear to be moving away from the people I love—and those who love or care about me?
- Treatment notwithstanding, do I seem more listless and lethargic than usual?

Regain a Sense of Hope and Control

Lack of hope can be a serious matter for you, because these feelings are often associated with depression. Untreated depression is one of the most significant factors impacting your cancer treatment and, in some situations, disease progression and survivorship. The question is, how do you maintain your sense of hope and control after a cancer diagnosis?

First of all, it's important to remember that every cancer has a recovery rate—so the outcome of your particular type of cancer isn't certain. Also, you must remember that help is available with stress-management techniques (see Chapter 8), by connecting with others whose lives have been impacted by cancer (see Chapter 14), by keeping up with your regular social contacts and interactions, by using hopeful and optimistic words about your life and relationships, and, most important, by changing your perspective and enjoying every moment as precious. No matter what, you can make plans for the future (the future involves any moment past this one). There's no reason not to do so!

Although no one can promise complete recovery, hope is there for the taking. According to Harold Benjamin, PhD, founder of The Wellness Community (now the Cancer Support Community), with hope comes an improved quality of life, which "is a reasonable goal itself."

Hope consists of three elements: a desire that an event will take place, the possibility that the event will occur, and the belief that you will be pleased if it does. Most important, hope is a thoughtful and rational process that begins with a realistic assessment of your situation—this is not just wishful thinking. No matter how dire the situation, hope embraces a decision to go forward irrespective of the outcome.

On the other hand, Dr. Benjamin said, hopelessness consists of only two elements: desire that an event will take place and the belief that no matter what you do, there is no possibility that the event will occur. "As you can see, hopelessness always includes a feeling of helplessness. In most cases of cancer, neither hopelessness nor helplessness is realistic, although the myths of cancer would fool you into thinking otherwise," he cautioned. "As a matter of fact, in the great majority of cases, it's unreasonable and unrealistic not to have hope."

Use Laughter as Medicine

Most of us are familiar with the old saying, "Laughter is the best medicine." One reason this phrase has stood the test of time is that it contains some truth. More and more research has shown the health benefits of laughter. A good laugh releases brain chemicals called endorphins, which lighten depression, reduce discomfort, and help in the healing process.

More than twenty-five years ago, before most experts understood the value of laughter in healing, Norman Cousins (a writer, author, and the longtime editor of Saturday Review) dealt with his own life-threatening illness by using laughter as a healing tool. He maintained a positive attitude and watched comedies—often, the Marx Brothers—daily on television and on tape. He laughed often and made sure to enjoy a hearty belly laugh several times each day.

All that laughter had its effect. Cousins's best-selling book, *Anatomy of an Illness as Perceived by the Patient*, reveals that the author's illness—plus a heart condition developed later—was kept at bay, perhaps even cured, by his regimen of positive emotions and laughter. Of course, there may have been other factors in his seemingly miraculous recovery, but Cousins's story is only one of many hailing the health benefits of laughter.

Gilda's Legacy of Love and Laughter

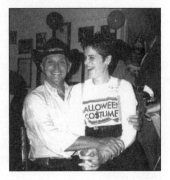

I stopped sitting at home saying, "Why me?" I began to crawl to The Wellness Community like someone in search of an oasis in the desert. My car couldn't get there fast enough to be nourished by other cancer patients and to know that I was not alone.

GILDA RADNER,
It's Always Something

Comedienne Gilda Radner, who came to The Wellness Community in Santa Monica when she was diagnosed with ovarian cancer, took a similar approach. Terminally ill, she still found much about which to laugh in life. She even wrote a book, *It's Always Something*, a frank description of living with cancer told in her inimitable humorous style. Radner's determination to continue being funny and to live fully for as long as possible has been an inspiration for tens of thousands of people who are living with cancer.

"When Gilda was first diagnosed, she withdrew from everyone," said Pam Zakheim, who grew up with Radner. "The difference between the day before she went to The Wellness Community and the day after her first visit was like night and day. Her hope was revitalized, as was her sense of self. She started communicating with her friends and family again. It was really quite inspiring."

Throughout the rest of her illness, Radner always remembered the lessons she had learned at The Wellness Community. "There will always be blood tests and X-rays and CAT scans and uncertainty," she said in her 1988 book. "The goal is to live a full, productive life, even with all that ambiguity. No matter what happens, whether the cancer never flares up again, or whether you die, the important thing is that the days that you have had, you will have LIVED. It's a hard concept, and it doesn't mean denying the depression and anger that come with cancer. But I've learned what I can control is whether I am going to live a day in fear and depression and panic, or whether I am going to attack the day and make it as good a day, as wonderful a day, as I can."

Join a Club . . . Just for Laughs

Laughing clubs were created in 1995 by Dr. Maden Kataria and his wife, Madhuri, of India. Today, these clubs are found worldwide (www.laughteryoga.org)—at health care centers, workplaces, assisted-living facilities, schools, senior centers, and health clubs—basically, anywhere people want more laughter. Groups meet weekly in some areas, and the only item on the agenda is to laugh.

So, it seems that guffaws and giggles are healthy in themselves for all of us, but they also serve as a way to keep cancer in its place. If cancer can't keep us from laughing and being ourselves in as many ways as possible, then we're not victims. After a cancer diagnosis, it's important to keep reminding yourself that you can still be YOU. Laughter is one of the tools that can help relieve stress—but it can also help you stay emotionally healthy throughout and beyond your treatment.

Gilda Radner and her husband, Gene Wilder, fully believed in the power of laughter as well. When Wilder and his friends Joel Siegel and Mandy Patinkin, along with Gilda's therapist Joanna Bull, set out to fulfill Gilda's wish that "no one should face cancer alone," they created the Gilda's Club program, which included many opportunities for laughter, and opened the first Clubhouse in New York City. Now that Gilda's Club Worldwide and The Wellness Community have merged to become the Cancer Support Community (CSC)—there are more opportunities for "laugh-ins" and other ways to connect with cancer survivors in a positive way worldwide.

Don't Blame Yourself

You aren't to blame for your illness, but in our society, too many individuals want to place blame somewhere. Many people, sadly, fault themselves for things that are truly beyond their control. Cancer is a good case in point.

Your lifestyle or some of the choices you've made can certainly weaken your immune system, but how can you be sure that's really what caused the cancer? Perhaps your immune system may be more susceptible to cancer cells than someone else's. You might have a genetic predisposition

to a certain disease, and it's possible that no preventative tactic or positive lifestyle choices would have made a difference.

The last thing you need in addition to your cancer is an unfair burden
of guilt. The Wellness Community's Dr. Benjamin said, "If you blame
yourself, you may trigger two other self-defeating reactions: You may
unconsciously forgo taking actions in your fight for recovery, and you
may inhibit the spontaneous self-healing responses your body would
automatically take to return to its normal condition."

So, give yourself a break. Deal with today's realities, not yesterday's
regrets. After all, today is all that any one of us truly has.

Patient Action Plan

- Acknowledge the change that cancer has brought to your
  life.
- Become informed.
- Get organized.
- Fight depression and hopelessness.
- Use laughter as medicine.
- Don't blame yourself.

Chapter 3

The Empowered Patient:
The Cancer Support Community Approach

People with cancer who participate in their recovery along with their health care team will improve the quality of their lives and may enhance the possibility of recovery. The "Patient Active'" concept combines the will of the patient with the skill of the physician—a powerful combination.

CANCER SUPPORT COMMUNITY'S "PATIENT ACTIVE" CONCEPT

I N 1982, The Wellness Community, founded by Dr. Harold Benjamin, provided an innovative comprehensive program of support based upon what he coined the "Patient Active" concept. The central belief, now supported by over thirty years of research by the Cancer Support Community (CSC) and others, is that people with cancer can adopt a set of actions, behaviors, and attitudes that can improve the quality of their lives and possibly enhance their recovery. By taking an active, rather than passive, approach to the illness, people can feel empowered, thus transforming the experience in a positive way, irrespective of the outcome of the disease.

Being an empowered patient is about active participation in the choices you make with your health care team. It's about being actively aware of the medical standard of care, new discoveries in cancer, and ways to manage side effects. It's about becoming involved in all aspects of your cancer experience and developing a new attitude toward the disease, treatment, and perhaps even life as a whole. Needless to say, in 1982, it was a revolutionary concept to believe that patients could actively partner with their physicians, let alone take specific actions that could help alleviate social and emotional pain from the illness and achieve better mental and physical outcomes.

Today, hundreds of thousands of people touched by cancer choose to be active participants and consumers in their cancer care.

Being empowered as a patient is not about one monumental decision, but rather a series of small, incremental choices. These choices help you regain a sense of control over your treatment and your life in general. There's no right or wrong way to act empowered, because, with this approach, you decide what's best for you. You can choose to make informed decisions about your own treatment, the management of your side effects, and the issues pertaining to your emotional and social well-being. This includes strengthening your relationships with others, as well as coping with the stress that cancer brings into your life. When you're motivated to take specific steps to help reduce feelings of loneliness, a loss of control, and a loss of hope, you will improve your quality of life.

Understand that you might feel overwhelmed right now and that the idea of acting empowered may seem foreign or too exhausting—that's okay. Take small steps. Engage as many supporters as possible to help you on this path. No one can make you empowered, and it will not happen overnight. Allow yourself time to feel vulnerable, as well as time to step up and take charge when you can.

In this book, we offer you information about advances in cancer treatment and emotional support—including support groups and other programs at CSC locations around the country or online at www .cancersupportcommunity.org. By addressing your intellectual, social, and emotional needs and by taking an active stance in your cancer care, you can get the most out of your cancer treatment and discover critical tools for your cancer journey.

An Empowered Patient

To be an Empowered Patient means that you aim to

- access resources for information and support;
- partner with your physician through open communication;
- make active choices in your treatment;
- develop a new attitude toward the illness and your life;
- make changes in your life that you think are important;
- regain a sense of control.

Form a Partnership with Your Physician

Because a good relationship with the right physician is critical if you wish to take a more active role in your care, it's important to focus time and energy on achieving such a relationship. A good partnership with your physician often includes open, direct communication and shared decision-making about the best treatment options for you. Here are some steps to get you on the road to a productive partnership with your physician.

- **Step One: Choose a medically competent physician.**
  In most cases, this is done by recommendation and reputation. There are also situations in which your insurance carrier or health-maintenance organization (HMO) will select your physician, ideally with some level of expertise in the type of cancer you have. Ask around. Talk to other cancer patients or your family doctor about what centers and physicians offer the best treatment options for your type of cancer.

- **Step Two: Ensure that the relationship is, at the very least, cordial.**
  It does not have to blossom into a full-blown friendship for it to be effective and efficient. It's only necessary that it be agreeable with open communication and that you feel you can understand each other. Know that it can take time to build rapport, but respect your intuition if it doesn't seem like a good fit.

- **Step Three: Make sure that you and your doctor clearly understand the expectations you have of each other.**
  Some patients want every bit of information and detail they can get, while others prefer to stick to the high points. Make sure that your doctor knows how much you want to know—and how much involvement you need in your treatment plan.

- **Step Four: If your needs as a patient conflict seriously with your doctor's, consider whether it's in your best interest to find another physician.**
  Many people find it embarrassing or difficult to leave a physician, but it is not unthinkable, nor should it be impossible. Talk with a

range of experienced doctors until you find one with whom you'd like to work. This is possibly the most serious medical situation you may have faced in your life. You need to feel confident in the relationship going forward.

- **Step Five: Find an advocate within your oncology-care team to coordinate your care.**
  Often, cancer patients are treated by a group of physicians that may include an *oncologist, radiologist, surgeon*, and/or another kind of specialist, along with the family doctor. A frequent complaint is that no one seems to be in charge—each physician acts almost independently, and there's no one from whom the patient can get all of the information he or she needs to make a decision. To be an empowered patient, we urge you to encourage one of the doctors to serve as coordinator of the team and keeper of all information. This should be your point person throughout treatment.

> *If I learned one thing, it's that when dealing with any chronic illness (like cancer) you have to be your own best advocate. Doctors aren't perfect. There were several times that we brought a second opinion to the table and Dan's doctor accepted it and worked with us. It can be very scary reading all of the medical literature, but in the end, we always felt better to be armed with information…versus just sitting back and letting someone else make the decisions. Being proactive with research and questioning allowed us to be more involved and helped remove some of the feelings of being totally out of control.*
>
> MEG,
> *caregiver*

The Cancer Support Community Patient/Oncologist Statement

As your physician, I will make every effort to:

- Provide you with personalized care that will, to the best of my knowledge, bring you the greatest benefit.
- Inform and educate you about your situation, and the various treatment alternatives. How detailed an explanation is given will be dependent upon your specific desires.

- Encourage you to ask questions about your illness and its treatment and answer your questions as clearly as possible. I will discuss your medical situation only with those people authorized by you.
- Remain aware that all major decisions about the course of your care will be made by you. However, I will accept the responsibility for making certain decisions if you want me to.
- Assist you in obtaining other professional opinions if you desire, or if I believe it to be in your best interest.
- Relate to you as one competent adult to another, always attempting to consider that your emotional, social, and psychological needs, as well as your physical needs, are all vital factors in your care.
- Honor appointment times unless an emergency arises and make all test results available promptly if you desire such reports.
- Return phone calls as promptly as possible, especially those you indicate as urgent.
- Enlist a team of nurses, office staff, and other professionals to help you manage the whole experience of cancer and its treatment.
- Provide you with any information you request concerning my training, experience, philosophy, and fees.
- Respect your desire to try treatment that might not be conventionally accepted. However, I will give you my honest opinion about such unconventional treatments.
- Maintain my active support and attention throughout the course of the illness.

As the patient, I will:

- Become informed to the best of my ability about my cancer and its treatment.
- Come prepared to appointments with a list of questions and concerns to discuss.
- Participate actively with you in developing a treatment plan that will bring me the greatest benefit, while respecting my life situation and goals.

- Adhere to the best of my ability with our mutually agreed-upon treatment plan.
- Be as candid as possible about what I need and expect from you and my medical team.
- Be honest about wanting or needing another professional opinion, as well as other forms of therapy in which I am involved including complementary or alternative therapies.
- Pursue activities and services that will help with my emotional, social, or practical needs so that these concerns do not get in the way of my treatment plan.
- Honor all appointment times unless an emergency arises.
- Be as considerate as possible when it comes to my doctor's need to be with other patients.
- Make all phone calls to my doctor during working hours. I will call at night or on weekends only when absolutely necessary.
- Coordinate the requests of my family and friends, so that all questions can be answered by my doctor at one time.

Treatment Decision-Making: A Critical Step

Many people are shocked after being diagnosed. For example, Abigail was bombarded with conflicting information after being diagnosed with cancer. She would lay awake mulling over questions as she waited to see a surgeon, but at her appointment, she froze and forgot to ask them. When the surgeon gave her information, she couldn't process it. Abigail ended up driving two hours each way from her farm during harvest season for radiation treatments. Later she felt she'd made a mistake. Had she been able to focus, she would have realized that the surgeon's recommendation for breast conservation didn't fit her priorities. She just agreed to what the doctor said without expressing her needs or understanding the consequences.

In a recent CSC survey of 1,022 breast cancer survivors, 52 percent said they had made a treatment decision at their first meeting with a cancer specialist, despite the fact that only 15 percent of these patients received information about their cancer before this visit. Approximately 34 percent indicated some "question regret." They lamented not knowing what to ask, or, like Abigail, forgetting to pose questions they had already formulated.

The truth is, many patients report feeling overwhelmed from the point of diagnosis on; they don't know what questions to ask their doctors or how to effectively use information given to them. Despite efforts to promote a culture of patient-centered care, it appears that many patients are not yet fully empowered to participate in the treatment decision-making process.

Open to Options™

Ask Questions, Gain Confidence, Be Empowered to Face Cancer

To fill this need, the CSC created a "decision-support" program called Open to Options™. A key feature of this program is to help patients develop a written list of questions that focuses on their personal goals and objectives for treatment that they can bring to appointments in which a treatment decision is to be made. Our research shows that patients who bring important questions with them experience more productive visits with their doctors. In fact, patients who learned how to focus on their key questions, goals, and objectives, had significantly less regret about treatment decisions they had made.

This program provides a research-proven framework using a model known as SCOPED (an acronym using the first letter of each kind of question). This model, developed by Dr. Jeff Belkora at the University of California, San Francisco, and further enhanced by the CSC, is now available as a free service to cancer patients nationwide through a toll-free call center. If you find yourself preparing for an upcoming treatment decision, call to schedule an appointment with one of our trained Open to Options™ specialists, who can help you write down what questions are most important to you.

The following is a sample list of questions in the SCOPED format and is not meant to be a comprehensive guide for each patient. You will determine which questions are right for you.

- **S**ituation (key facts and knowledge gaps): **What questions or concerns do you have about your situation?**
  What type or stage of cancer do I have?
  What do my test and pathology reports say?
  How serious is this?

As a single parent, will I be able to care for my children on my own?

- **C**hoices (available options): **What questions do you have about the treatment choices available to you?**
  What are my treatment options? What are the different side effects with each treatment?
  How much time do I have to make a treatment decision?
  Do I need more tests?
  Are there any clinical trials that would be best for my type of cancer?
  Where can I go for treatment?
  Will my insurance cover the costs involved in a clinical trial? Up to what extent?

- **O**bjectives: **What are my goals or concerns for treatment or for this visit?**
  What are my priorities? Hopes? Fears? Thoughts or feelings?
  What are the goals of treatment?
  How much detail can I handle?
  What's the timeline? What do I want?

- **P**eople (roles and responsibilities): **What questions or concerns do I have about the roles and responsibilities of people involved in my care?**
  What are my specific preferences for my doctor's involvement (e.g., give information, make a recommendation, make decisions for me)?
  What are the roles and responsibilities of other people involved in my care?
  Where else can I go for advice, information, or support? Is there a Cancer Support Community or other support program nearby? How do I locate a program in my area?

- **E**valuation (impact of choices on objectives): **What questions do I have about how my choices might affect my goals and concerns?**

How will my choices affect my survival, possible recurrence, and
  my quality of life?

- **D**ecisions (best choices and next steps)
  Have I already made any decisions?
  Am I leaning toward any specific choices?
  What else do I need to know to arrive at a decision I feel comfort-
    able with and can follow through?

Patient Action Plan

The following tips are designed to help you prepare for each
doctor's visit and to build trust and confidence with your doctor
and your treatment decisions.

- **Strive to be an Empowered Patient.**
  Regain a sense of control, support, and hope.
- **Bring along the list of questions that you've prepared for
  your doctor.**
  Use the *Open to Options*™ model (described above). Send your
  questions in advance to your doctor or provide them at the start of
  your visit to ensure that your questions get asked—and answered.
- **Prepare a written list of other issues you want your doctor to
  know.**
  These can include how you've been feeling or what you hope
  to achieve. Bring the list with you, so that you don't forget to
  share information about your health and emotional state.
- **If you don't understand something your doctor says, ask for
  clarification.**
  If you still don't understand, ask again, or ask the nurse to
  explain it further.
- **Take someone with you when you go to the doctor.**
  Your family member or trusted ally might be able to listen to
  and understand the doctor with greater objectivity. If someone
  cannot attend, ask if you can audio-record the session.
- **Get a second opinion.**
  If a major course of action is being discussed, a second
  opinion is very important.

- **Most importantly, adhere as closely as possible with the treatment plan that you agree upon with your physician.** If you're not able to do what your doctor is advising, then ask yourself: "Why not?" Perhaps you need to have further discussions with your doctor right away.

We encourage you to create a partnership with your health care team. As one patient shared, "It's like we're flying a ship and together we are pilot and co-pilot. That gives me such great comfort, and I feel I'm in safe, supportive hands!"

Part Two

Knowing Your Options

Chapter 4

Getting a Second Opinion— and Maybe a Third

I've found a lot of people don't know anything about how to get a second opinion and how meaningful it can be. I always tell people to go to a teaching hospital that specializes in cancer—or, better yet, a melanoma center. Even if you have to travel out of state, it is ideal to get a different point of view from that of your local doctor.

Liz,
melanoma survivor

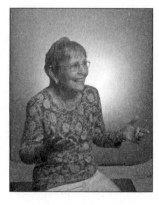

aLL CANCERS are best treated when they are diagnosed early. There are many types of cancer, so it's crucial that the disease be diagnosed accurately and promptly. Treatment options depend upon careful identification of the type and stage of your cancer.

Because a biopsy is key to the diagnosis, it's important that you receive the appropriate type of biopsy and that the tissue sample is evaluated by a pathologist (a doctor who specializes in studying disease through the evaluation of body tissue). If your local doctor or hospital doesn't see many cancer patients, or if you have a rare kind of cancer, you might also need to seek out a comprehensive cancer center designated by the National Cancer Institute (NCI) or an academic medical center to ensure that you have access to a qualified pathologist.

Feeling confident that you are receiving the best treatment for your cancer is vitally important. Even if you have good communication with your physician and are comfortable with his or her qualifications, it's often useful to seek a second—or even third—opinion at various points along the way to be certain that you are being offered the best medical treatment possible. Keep in mind that some insurance programs even require second opinions, and many will cover such a cost if the patient requests one (see Chapter 10).

Most doctors expect and understand that because of the serious nature of cancer, patients will seek a second opinion. Don't be afraid that you will hurt your doctor's feelings, or that he or she will treat you differently. A good doctor will be respectful of your need to confirm that you are getting the best available treatment.

Consider having your consultation in a multidisciplinary setting at a major cancer center or university hospital, if possible. Some of the particular circumstances when you might want to seek another opinion are

- you want to be sure that you're on the right course;
- there's something vague about your case, such as whether or not a tumor is operable;
- you live in a rural area and are getting treatment at a small hospital;
- you're on a managed care plan that you feel is limiting your treatment options;
- you've been told that there is no hope and no further treatment that can be of benefit.

In seeking another qualified opinion, your doctor will appreciate that you're gathering vital information that will help both of you make even more informed decisions about your treatment.

Don't be afraid to say to your doctor, "I don't like that."

CINDY,
colorectal cancer survivor

Finding a Specialist

Cancer is a complex and challenging disease. The way of classifying and treating cancer can change quickly. Oncologists are doctors who specialize in cancer. Often a patient diagnosed with cancer will see a variety of specialists: a surgeon, a radiologist, or an oncologist specializing in the type of cancer diagnosed.

Your primary doctor or your insurance company can often recommend an oncologist or cancer specialist to you for a first or second opinion. If you do seek another doctor's opinion, remember that it's best to have a complete copy of your medical records, including original X-rays, pathology slides, and medical reports on hand. Ask for copies of all tests as you take them, and keep them in a personal folder.

You'll probably want to seek care from a cancer specialist who is a member of a professional society, such as the American Society of Clinical Oncology (ASCO), the American Association for Cancer Research (AACR), and/or the American Society of Hematology (ASH). These organizations are dedicated to improving the treatment of cancer, as well as preventing and curing the disease. A specialist will most likely be on the cutting edge of cancer care by reading articles and attending scientific meetings about the newest treatments for cancer. If possible, consult with a specialist who's

> *A second opinion is not considered adequate unless another pathologist, preferably a cancer expert, reviews the actual tissue sample of the tumor itself.*

connected with a multidisciplinary cancer center or a university hospital known for cancer research. Comprehensive cancer centers that are some of the best places in the country to receive cancer treatment are listed on the Web site of the NCI (http://cancercenters.cancer.gov).

Making Sense of the Numbers

The effectiveness of treatment can be seen "in the numbers," meaning the statistics, but be wary of letting statistics distress you and rule your life. Remember: You're more than a number—and you aren't a statistic. Your experience with cancer is unique and might vary greatly from statistics that represent large populations of cancer patients.

Cancer survival statistics are based on five-year survival rates. Five-year survival can—and does—happen for many people with all stages of many cancer types. As a rule, you have the best odds for long-term survival if you're diagnosed with early-stage disease. As the stage increases, the chance of long-term survival is reduced. Many new treatments, however, make it possible to manage or even control later stages of certain types of cancer for a long period of time, which is another good reason to obtain several medical opinions.

Dealing with Conflicting Advice

If you receive a recommendation that's different from the original treatment plan proposed to you, you'll most likely be confused. You should discuss why the plans are different with both doctors. For some types of cancer, there might be multiple treatment options, many of which are equally effective. This is an important time to ask questions that will help you determine what to do and to consider how the various options will impact your lifestyle. Because so much is at stake, you might feel that you need a third opinion.

Remember, getting a second or third opinion does not mean that you have to change your treatment course or find a new doctor. Use the information to discuss what treatment options are right for you with your initial oncologist. Many people have shared that they feel better and more in control after they've talked to another expert about their disease. As they proceed with treatment, they feel more confident that they've explored every possible option to receive the best available care.

No "Magic Cure"

Keep in mind that going from doctor to doctor searching for a "magic cure" is not necessarily productive for your disease or your mental health. Some patients make it even harder on themselves by getting opinion after opinion and then feeling immobilized because they can't figure out what to do. If that's happening to you or someone you know, talk to your physician, an oncology social worker, or a nurse to explore some of the fears and anxieties that you might have about making decisions, about starting or ending treatment, or about finding the right treatment team for you.

In some cases, you might not hear what you want to hear, no matter how many doctors you see. Be wary of any person who offers a quick or easy "cure" that doesn't seem consistent with any of the other medical professionals with whom you've discussed your case or treatment plan.

> *I like to be an active part of all the decisions that are made and be completely informed about what the doctors are doing. I take a lot of time to do my own research. I even bring things to their attention, to see if it's something they're willing to try.*
>
> ERICA,
> *colorectal cancer patient*

The Proactive Doctor Interview

Whether this is for a first, second, or third opinion, here are some effective questions to ask the doctors involved in your cancer diagnosis and/or treatment.

• How much experience do you have in cancer and in treating cancer?
• Specifically, are you board certified as an oncologist or hematologist or other specialty?
• How do you stay up to date on the latest cancer treatments?
• Are cancer clinical trials offered at this clinic/hospital?
• Where will my cancer treatment be provided?
• Are you, or the clinic, associated with a comprehensive cancer center, medical school, or major medical center?
• Will you and/or the hospital accept my type of insurance?
• Is there an oncology nurse or social worker available during my treatment for education and support?
• What other support services (support groups, housing, etc.) are available?

I learned from having cancer that you have to take care of yourself—if something doesn't feel right, do something about it. It made me "Patient Active." Now I tell my doctors what I want them to do for me.

MARILYN,
colorectal cancer survivor

Communicate with Your Health Care Team

Finding out that you have cancer can be frightening and overwhelming. It can make talking and listening to your doctor, nurse, other members of your health care team, and even your family very difficult. Fortunately, there are several strategies you can use to make communicating with your doctor easier. Studies show that clear communication between you and your health care team can help you feel better about your choices and might even improve the quality of your care.

Make sure that you understand what is being discussed. When you talk with your doctor, use "I" statements. For example, the phrase "I don't understand…" is much more effective than "You're being unclear about…" Also, be assertive. If you don't understand a word or a treatment option, say so. Make your questions specific and brief. If there's something you don't understand, ask your doctor to discuss it in more detail. Write down your questions and concerns.

Finally, if something seems confusing, try repeating it back to your doctor in this way: "You mean I should…" If you think you'll understand better with pictures, ask to see X-rays or slides, or have the doctor draw a diagram.

To ensure that you are getting the absolute best care and treatment, you need to be as actively involved with your health care team as possible. Taking all of the best information from all of the best medical minds can go a long way toward a more positive and successful outcome.

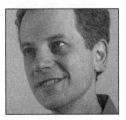

When I was first diagnosed with lung cancer, I was too overwhelmed and emotional to evaluate the options on my own. So I asked my brother and two other friends (all physicians) to serve as my "medical advisory team." It was important to have information processed for me in a way that I could deal with.

JERRY,
lung cancer survivor

Patient Action Plan

- **Always get at least one second opinion.**
  Two informed opinions are mandatory, regarding your cancer diagnosis or treatment.
- **Talk to your doctor about your goals and objectives for treatment.**
  This includes the possibility and appropriateness of a cancer clinical trial.
- **Keep a file of your medical records on hand.**
  Request copies of all relevant tests—including reports about your surgery, pathology reports, and radiology reports—from

any physician with whom you are consulting. Call before your appointment to make sure the physician's office received all of the necessary information prior to your visit.

- **Bring a family member or close friend to appointments to take notes.**
  A companion can help ask questions and provide you with emotional support.
- **Consider recording the conversation with permission from your physician.**
  Recording your consultation will help you review important information after the appointment.

Remember, though there may not be a "magic cure" for your cancer, it helps to weigh the pros and cons of input from many experienced and knowledgeable physicians.

Chapter 5

Evaluating Traditional Treatment Options

It is your job to jump in and find what you can find—there are re- sources out there. You have to go out and look for where all that support is, taking names, kicking doors. It's not going to come easily.

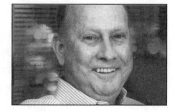

CARL,
multiple myeloma survivor

REATMENT FOR ALL TYPES of cancer is improving rapidly, and it's often hard to determine the best treatment to use if you are giv- en multiple options. It's important to gather as much information as you can about your options and ask any and all questions. Medical decisions are ultimately yours to make in partnership with your health care team; this is your body and your life—so you have ultimate control over these decisions.

Before you make a treatment decision, talk with your doctor about how each treatment works to stop the cancer; the possible side effects for each option; and what practical things you will have to consider, such as transportation to treatment, time commitment, and cost. When you feel ready, you'll have to determine if a certain therapy is worth taking when you consider how it will impact your lifestyle and your ultimate goal for the therapy.

It might be valuable to get a second, or even third, opinion with on- cology experts before making a decision. It's also important to ask your doctor about new developments in the treatment of your cancer, includ- ing targeted therapies (see Chapter 6) or whether a clinical trial would be an option for you (see Chapter 7).

Overall, being proactive is especially critical when you're making treatment decisions. You should remember that you have time to learn everything you can about your options and about the treatments available to you. Take a deep breath, and take time to seek information and advice. Ask questions, and then do what is right for you.

Chemotherapy

Chemotherapy is the use of drugs to destroy cancer cells. Estimates suggest that up to half of all cancer patients receive chemotherapy. Chemotherapeutic drugs kill rapidly growing cells—cancer cells and nearby healthy cells. Because these drugs affect the healthy cells, side effects such as fatigue, diarrhea, peripheral neuropathy, and others are common. These side effects can delay scheduled treatments or result in decreased chemotherapy drug doses. Many side effects are temporary, can be controlled or managed (see Chapter 9), and stop once treatment has been completed or stopped. The type of chemotherapy given depends upon the type of cancer, the stage of cancer, and your overall health. There are many different types of "chemo" drugs available, but, generally, you and your oncologist will discuss a specific treatment plan (or protocol) that's considered the standard of care for your cancer in its present form.

One of the most important things to consider with chemotherapy is that, when possible, it's important to "stay the course." Unnecessary changes or delays in your chemotherapy treatment schedule can negatively impact outcomes. It's very important that you report all symptoms or side effects to your doctor and/or nurse so that they can be treated effectively.

How Chemotherapy Has Changed

In the past, chemotherapy was synonymous with debilitating side effects. Today, more effective drugs in higher doses and combinations have been developed to improve the possibility of long-term survivorship, while reducing the side effects of treatment for many cancers.

How Chemotherapy Is Administered

Generally, chemotherapy is administered in an outpatient setting, on a regular schedule, and for a limited period of time. You might receive a combination or sequence of drugs proven to be most effective.

Chemotherapy might be given intravenously (by vein), in pill form (by mouth), through an injection (shot), or applied directly on the skin.

It's important to ask specific questions about what treatments you'll need and what to expect in the weeks and months ahead. You'll want to track your treatment schedule and follow-up appointments in your calendar and keep a journal of your side effects and experiences so you can stay on schedule, manage problems, and take an active role in your care.

> *After you understand your condition completely and decide upon a treatment, do not spend a lot of time second-guessing the doctors or other treatment options. Feel empowered that you made the best decision with the information you know.*
>
> MELANOMA SURVIVOR

Dose Is Key

In one recent study, an ongoing review of medical charts for more than 17,000 women receiving chemotherapy with early-stage breast cancer showed these results.

- Up to 20 percent of patients were receiving less than 85 percent of the planned chemotherapy dose. Data suggests that without the proper dose intensity, the risk for cancer relapse is much greater, and the overall survival rate is reduced.
- The most common reason for reduced dose intensity, or for treatments to be rescheduled, is low white blood cell counts. Low counts lead to higher risks of infection—a preventable condition, if treated proactively.

How Does Chemotherapy Work?

Cancer cells divide and multiply uncontrollably, while normal cells grow and die in a controlled way. Chemotherapy drugs destroy cancer cells by stopping them from growing and multiplying. Because chemotherapy is a "systemic" treatment, it kills any rapidly dividing cell in its path. Healthy cells can also be harmed, especially those that divide quickly, which is what causes many of the side effects people expect from chemotherapy, such as hair loss or nausea. The kind of side effects experienced depends on the kind of drugs you get, the doses, and the frequency of treatments. Previously healthy cells usually repair themselves after treatment is over, but it's important that you actively manage any side effects when you experience them.

Goals of Chemotherapy

Depending on the type of cancer and how advanced it is, chemotherapy can be used for different goals.

- **Goal 1: Cure the cancer.**
  Cancer is considered cured when the patient remains free of any evidence of measurable tumor on physical examination or laboratory and radiology studies.
- **Goal 2: Control the cancer.**
  Control is keeping the cancer from spreading, slowing the cancer's growth, and killing cancer cells that might have spread to other parts of the body from the original tumor.
- **Goal 3: Relieve symptoms that the cancer may be causing.**
  Relieving symptoms such as pain and discomfort can help patients live more comfortably.

Radiation Treatment

Radiation treatment, also referred to as radiotherapy or radiation therapy, is the use of high-energy X-rays to stop cancer cells from growing and multiplying. High-energy beams are aimed directly at the location of your cancer by an X-ray machine that is a radiation source. Nearly half of all people with cancer are treated with radiation. For many patients, radiation is the only kind of treatment needed.

Radiation therapy is given in divided doses (measured in rads or grays), usually five days a week for several weeks. You'll work very closely with the radiation oncologist and a highly skilled group of radiation technicians and nurses who will support you with high-tech, high-quality care.

Prior to radiation, precise measurements will be taken of exactly where the radiotherapy is to be given. The technicians will draw special markings on your skin to guide them—and the machine—in giving you effective treatment. You will not be radioactive during this time, and, generally, you won't feel anything during the treatment itself, except perhaps a little discomfort from lying still for a period of time. Many people are able to arrange their daily radiation appointments around work or other daily activities. Sometimes the best time to go is early in the morning; that way, you have your whole day to be active.

Another kind of radiation treatment involves internal radiation; an exact amount of radioactive material is implanted inside your body, usually as treatment for cancer of the cervix, prostate, or breast. The implant is left in place for a few days. During that time, you'll generally stay in the hospital while the radioactive implant works to destroy the tumor.

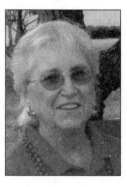

Years ago, before my first cancer diagnosis, I dreaded ever getting hit with the information that I had breast cancer. After my first experience, which was a lumpectomy and radiation, I found that I was able to basically return to my normal life. That which I had feared was survivable.

NANCY HUTCHINS,

participant, Cancer Support Community, Central New Jersey

Goals of Radiation Therapy

The goal of radiation therapy depends on the type of cancer and how advanced it is.

- **Goal 1: Shrink the tumor.**
  Radiation can be an important tool to stop the growth of cancer cells that remain after surgery or to reduce the size of a tumor before surgery.
- **Goal 2: Improve quality of life.**
  Even when curing the cancer isn't possible, radiation therapy can still bring relief. Many patients find that symptoms, such as pain, are greatly improved with radiotherapy.

Doctors do half the work in healing, and we have to do the other half: healing emotions and spirit.

DIANA BERHO,
community member, Cancer Support Community, Redondo Beach

Surgery

Surgery can be used in the diagnosis, staging (which describes the severity), and treatment of cancer. In early stages of cancer, surgery alone can be used to remove the cancer and cure the body. It has played a major role in the cure of early stage melanoma as well as breast, colorectal, and thyroid cancers. Surgery alone can be curative in patients with localized disease, but it's often necessary to combine surgery with other treatments such as chemotherapy, radiation, or targeted therapy (see Chapter 6) to achieve higher response rates. Surgery can also be used to minimize the symptoms of advanced disease, to relieve distress, or for reconstructive and rehabilitative purposes.

A biopsy is the surgical removal of a tissue sample from an organ or other part of the body (usually from a tumor) for examination by a pathologist. Most people have a biopsy to confirm or diagnose cancer correctly. A positive biopsy indicates the presence of cancer, and a negative biopsy can indicate either that no cancer is present or that the biopsy specimen was inadequate.

A common, unproven myth is that surgery can cause cancer to spread by exposing the cancerous cells to air. This just isn't true. Cancer doesn't spread because it's been exposed to air. However, some patients feel worse after surgery than they did before, due to discomfort from the incision and anesthesia. This feeling is absolutely normal. Because early removal of all cancer cells provides the best chance of a cure, it's important that you not allow this myth to discourage you from seeking surgery.

Goals of Surgery

Depending on the type of cancer and how advanced it is, surgery can be used for different goals.

- **Goal 1: Prevent cancer.**
  In some cases, surgery can prevent cancer before it begins. Examples include the removal of precancerous polyps in

the rectum or colon to prevent colorectal cancer or having a prophylactic mastectomy to prevent breast cancer where there is a high genetic and hereditary risk.

- **Goal 2: Diagnose and stage the cancer.**
  Surgery can identify the tumor type, extent of growth, size, nodal involvement, and regional and/or distant spread.
- **Goal 3: Cure.**
  The primary goal of cancer surgery is to cure. Definitive or curative surgery involves removing the entire tumor, associated lymph nodes, and a 2- to 5-centimeter margin of surrounding tissue. To increase the likelihood of a cure, early detection is essential.
- **Goal 4: Relieve symptoms.**
  Surgery can be used to minimize symptoms of advanced disease, such as neurosurgical procedures for pain control.
- **Goal 5: Reconstruct or rehabilitate.**
  The goal is to minimize deformity and improve quality of life (as with breast, head, and neck reconstruction).

I got all of my tests, reports, and biopsy results and kept copies so that I could read everything and go back over it. I think that's very important. No one can remember it all.

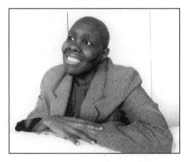

CYNTHIA,
community member, Cancer Support Community, Greater St. Louis

Targeted Therapies

Targeted therapies are new approaches to cancer treatment that aim to "target" certain cellular characteristics found only in cancer cells (and not in normal cells). The idea is that targeted therapies only kill cancerous cells, leaving healthy cells unharmed. More information about these exciting treatments is found in Chapter 6.

The Cancer Support Community Treatment Decision-Making Tool

We've recommended that you construct a question list to prepare for doctors' visits. The following question-and-answer chart is also helpful for the discussion of treatment options with your doctor. Fill this out and bring it to your appointment as a guide to help you make treatment decisions.

PART ONE

Medical Background Questions	Answers
When was I diagnosed? (A person with newly diagnosed cancer may have different treatment options than a person who has already had certain treatments.)	
What type of cancer do I have? (The type of cancer will determine the type of treatment you need.)	
What is the stage of my cancer? (The stage of the cancer will also determine the types of treatments available.)	
What is my current health status? (Your overall health status may affect the types of treatments you can tolerate.)	
What is the goal of my treatment? (The goal of treatment—cure, symptom control, prolonged remission—may affect the type of treatment that is available to you or that you select.)	

PART TWO

Treatment Options	As you discuss treatment options with your doctor, take notes under each column below.		
YOU HAVE CHOICES!	Potential Side Effects (hospitalization, fatigue, peripheral neuropathy, nausea and vomiting, rash, hair loss, etc.)	Quality of Life/ Treatment Convenience (required visits to the hospital or clinic to receive treatment, monitoring, blood counts, restricting activities, etc.)	Effectiveness (What are the chances that this treatment will work for me?)
Surgery (Can the tumor be surgically removed?)			
Pre- or Post-Surgery Chemotherapy			
Pre- or Post-Surgery Radiation			
Radiation			
Chemotherapy			
Targeted Therapies			
Investigational Therapies in Clinical Trials			
Combination Treatments			
Best Supportive Care			

Patient Action Plan

- **Carefully weigh the treatment options presented to you.**
  Be proactive in gathering information and getting second
  opinions about your treatment options.
- **Bring someone with you to medical appointments.**

Emotional support helps you hear what's being said so you can discuss it together later.

- **Ask practical questions.**
  Where and how often will you receive treatment? Will you have follow-up visits with the doctor in-between treatment appointments, or will you need to make additional appointments for labs before treatment days? Will all costs be covered by insurance, or will you incur out-of-pocket costs?
- **Know which physical side effects to expect and the strategies to prevent or treat them.**
  Fatigue, hair loss, nausea, fever, and infection are common side effects.
- **Throughout treatment, keep a question list and write down how you feel between visits.**
  Keeping track of how you feel will help enhance conversations with your doctor or oncology nurse.
- **Talk to your physician or oncology nurse about any anxiety you have regarding treatment.**
  It may help to consider stress-reduction exercises, meditation, or medication.
- **Consider making an appointment with a social worker or counselor.**
  Or join a support group with others who are going through cancer treatment. Such support can help you and your family prepare for emotional and social issues.
- **Contact a cancer support organization.**
  The Cancer Support Community (www .cancersupportcommunity.org) is one organization that can provide you with more information or help you find others in your area who have been through similar experiences and can offer guidance.
- **Set goals and rewards for yourself as you reach treatment milestones.**
- **Know that you always have options.**

Chapter 6

New Frontiers in Treatment

SURGERY, CHEMOTHERAPY, and radiation remain the standard ways to treat cancer, but we look forward to the day when cancer treatment can be tailored to each individual—and a day when the word "cure" is more a part of our vocabulary. While cancer treatment is not yet at that point, scientists have made great advances in medical research, bringing us much closer to the goal of personalizing medicine.

Over the past decade, great advances have been made in understanding the differences between cancer cells and normal cells. Because of this, researchers have been able to make remarkable progress in

- developing drugs that can target cancer cells without affecting healthy cells, often called targeted therapies;
- biomarker screening for specific elements of cancer cells that can be used to individualize treatment.

Tailoring, or personalizing, medicine involves new tests and techniques that help doctors understand more about each person's cancer at the cellular level. When a physician knows more about a patient's actual cancer cells, he or she can select drugs and treatments that will more likely lead to a successful outcome with fewer harmful side effects. This is the future: a future where doctors can know more about what's happening in your body and where cancer treatments will be more effective at finding and correcting problems.

Starting at the Cellular Level

Cancer is a genetic disease, meaning that it starts with gene mutations or changes within cells. Genetic disease is different from hereditary disease, which involves a family connection to a disease such as cancer. In all cases, cancer cells are created when the genetic material (DNA) that controls the cell life cycle is damaged and a mutated cell called "cancer" is formed. In other words, not everyone has a hereditary connection to cancer, but everyone who has had cancer has had a genetic mutation that caused it.

Within the cell's DNA, genes make specific proteins required for proper cell functioning; enzymes and receptors are examples of proteins found in a cell. When proteins do not function the way they're supposed to, they can cause cells to grow uncontrollably to form a tumor. Cancer research is focusing on the role of gene malfunctions in causing cancer. Scientists believe that comprehensive research in this area will provide the most promise for finding cures.

So far, scientists have identified many gene malfunctions that cause abnormal proteins that cannot perform their normal function at all or that cannot be controlled when they do their jobs. The three main gene groups being studied for the development of new cancer treatments at this time are: oncogenes, tumor suppressor genes, and DNA repair genes.

- Oncogenes produce abnormal proteins that cause cells to grow out of control and divide too quickly.
- Tumor suppressor genes normally restrict the rate of cell division. They promote apoptosis: a normal process by which cells self-destruct when they are too old or have become damaged. (Apoptosis is sometimes called "programmed cell death.") If these genes do not function properly, a tumor can develop.
- DNA repair genes repair the occasional mutations that normally develop in DNA during the process of cell division, but these genes can become mutated, in which case they cannot do their job of repairing mutations.

These and other genes involved with the formation of cancer cells are assumed to hold the key to information about which specific targets, at the molecular level, should be identified for drug development.

> Six years ago, I began to have pain in my lower back, and a CT scan showed a three-centimeter tumor on my kidney. After three opinions, we chose to do chemo (VCP) for six weeks and then Rituxan. The Rituxan was easily tolerated, and, within eight months, all

visible tumors had gone. To date, I still get nodes that appear and disappear on their own. I know I have cancer, but I feel that by being fit and eating well, my cancer remains under control.

MATTHEW ACCARDO,
community member, Cancer Support Community, Redondo Beach

Targeting Cancer Drugs to Cancer Cells

Unlike traditional therapies, new cancer treatments recognize cellular characteristics that distinguish cancer cells from normal cells. Doctors can use screening tests to identify the cancer cells in your body that would be susceptible to targeted treatments. The two main types of targeted therapies currently available are

- monoclonal antibodies;
- small molecule inhibitors.

Therapeutic Monoclonal Antibodies

Monoclonal antibodies (MABs or MoAbs) are antibodies created in the laboratory that target specific proteins (antigens) on the surface of cancer cells. (The generic drug names of monoclonal antibodies often end in "mab.")

When a monoclonal antibody binds with the protein antigen on cancer cells, it acts like a key that fits only one lock on the cell surface. Once a monoclonal antibody in a cancer drug locks into the cell's surface, one of several actions can occur to kill cancer cells.

- The monoclonal antibody can block signals to the core of the cancer cell (nucleus), so that it can no longer grow or repair itself.
- The monoclonal antibody can attract the body's immune system to destroy the cancer cell, or start the signal for cell death.

Scientists have discovered that monoclonal antibodies can also be used as a delivery system to take other treatment agents to cancer cells directly. For example, monoclonal antibodies are used to deliver radiation, chemotherapy, cytokines (immune system messengers), DNA molecules, and small molecule inhibitors to selectively targeted cells. Once the monoclonal antibody carries the other drug directly to the cancer, the drug can work to destroy the abnormal cells while leaving healthy cells unaffected.

To date, all versions of monoclonal antibody therapies are similar in their effectiveness and safety. Some people experience allergic reactions to this treatment, but that is treatable. Mostly, the potential benefits for cancer treatment are promising.

Small Molecule Inhibitors

Small molecule inhibitors (sometimes called enzyme inhibitors) inter-fere with signals inside the cell, to stop those signals from making the cancer cells grow and divide. The generic drug names of small molecule inhibitors often end in "inib."

In cancer cells, there is often an abnormally high level of signals instructing tumor cells to grow and divide faster than normal. Small molecule inhibitors block the actions of the enzyme-growth receptors and prevent cell-growth signals from reaching the nucleus of the cancer cells. In this way, they are able to prevent cancer cells from dividing.

What Are the "Targets" for Anti-Cancer Drugs?

A good target for a cancer drug is one known to affect the growth and survival of cancer cells. There are many signaling pathways in cancer cells that promote cell division by activating a specific receptor on the cell wall. Scientists have begun to successfully develop drugs that block some of these pathways.

Two examples of targets that fall into this category belong to a fam-ily of protein receptors found on the surface of normal and cancer cells called human epidermal growth factor receptors (EGFR). There are at least four members of this family of receptors: HER1, HER2, HER3, and HER4. Doctors sometimes refer to HER1 as "EGFR," because this was the first receptor found. Later, other members of the HER family were found, which is why the numeric distinction was applied.

Scientists have found that many types of cancer cells have high levels of HER1 (EGFR) or HER2. When abnormally high levels of these pro-teins are present on the cell surface, cells divide too rapidly, thus caus-ing cancer tumors. Specific tests can measure whether abnormal levels of HER1 (EGFR) or HER2 are present in tissue samples. Patients can then be treated with anti-cancer drugs that block, or inhibit, HER1- or HER2-related tumor growth, including: Herceptin® (trastuzumab), a

monoclonal antibody used against breast cancer; Tarceva® (erlotin.
a small molecule drug used against non-small cell lung cancer or advanced pancreatic cancer; or Erbitux® (cetuximab) a monoclonal antibody used against colorectal cancer or certain types of head and neck
cancer. These drugs target human epidermal growth factor receptors to
stop the related cancer cells from dividing.

Another important target for anti-cancer therapies is the vascular endothelial growth factor (VEGF). VEGF is a protein that stimulates growth and
is necessary for the production of the blood vessels in cancerous tumors.
Without these vessels, tumors have difficulty growing because they are otherwise starved of nutrients. VEGF is produced naturally by the body, but
can also be produced in abnormal amounts by cancer cells. VEGF becomes
an important biomarker for cancer diagnosis and treatment.

Antiangiogenesis agents are a class of drugs that target VEGF to
starve cancerous tumors. Angiogenesis is the normal biologic process
of developing new blood vessels that transport nutrients and oxygen
to cells and organs. During the development and spread of cancer, this
process works against the body, because tumors use the same process
to feed their growth. New blood vessels may "feed" cancer cells with
oxygen and nutrients, allowing the bad cells to grow, move into nearby
tissue, and spread to other parts of the body.

Scientists are determining ways to reverse or stop the process of angiogenesis. Selectively cutting off or "starving" the growth system of tumor
cells is called antiangiogenesis. One example of a drug that falls into this
category is Avastin® (bevacizumab), a monoclonal antibody used to treat
metastatic colorectal cancer, metastatic non-small cell lung cancer, metastatic breast cancer, glioblastoma, and metastatic kidney cancer.

There are several other examples of targeted therapies that are available to treat different kinds of cancers. A complete list and discussion of
anti-cancer drugs currently available in the United States can be found
on the National Cancer Institute (NCI) Web site (www.cancer.gov/
cancertopics/factsheet/Therapy/targeted).

Targeted treatments may work better when they are used in combination with cell-killing agents such as

- radioactive isotopes;
- chemotherapy drugs;
- toxins.

ₗ 59

nations allow the cell-killing drug or radioactivity to be
y to the cancer cell, with the goal of sparing normal,

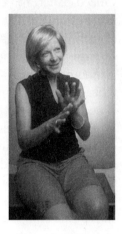

*᷈ce I got up-to-date information about my
type of melanoma, learned about my treatment options, and identified an expert oncologist and surgeon, it was easier to make
decisions. That's when I felt less stressed.*

CINDY,
melanoma survivor

Cancer Vaccines

Stimulating the body's immune system, also known as immunotherapy,
has been studied by cancer researchers for many years. Because cancer
cells are "insiders" and have a mechanism to help make them invisible
to the body's immune system, cancer cells can multiply into large tumors without triggering an effective immune response. Cancer vaccines
are being developed to counter these tactics by tricking the immune
system into recognizing the tumor and prompting the immune system
to fight back.

Cancer vaccines have several proven and potential advantages over
standard therapies.

- **They are well tolerated, with few and fairly minor side effects.**
  This is because they help the immune system distinguish if cells
  are tumor or normal cells, so that only harmful cells will be attacked. Standard therapy kills both tumor cells and healthy cells,
  causing unpleasant—and sometimes serious—side effects.

- **They may produce longer remissions or prevent recurrence.**
  Once the immune system is triggered to attack tumor cells, it might
  remain on alert longer to destroy them. With standard therapy, a
  few resistant tumor cells are often able to survive and cause a return of the disease.

- They may be effective even against metastatic disease—cancer that has spread beyond its initial site to other parts of the body. The immune system serves the entire body and can hunt down and destroy wandering tumor cells wherever they gather.

Many cancer vaccines are undergoing clinical trials to evaluate their effectiveness. In 2010, the first therapeutic cancer vaccine called Provenge® (sipuleucel-T) was approved by the Food and Drug Administration (FDA) for the treatment of prostate cancer. The promising research in this area is offering a great deal of hope for researchers and patients alike.

Recruiting the Immune System (Immunotherapy)

Continued research into better strategies for stimulating the body's immune system to fight cancer is ongoing. For example, one area of immunotherapy research is with the use of cytokines, which are considered "immune system messengers." Some cytokines, which can be produced in the laboratory, can be given to patients to either boost their own immune systems or to slow down the growth of the cancer.

Another immunotherapy research strategy involves adoptive immunotherapy, which genetically instructs a human immune cell to seek and kill cancer cells. Cells called T-cells are taken from a patient and modified; when they are returned to the patient, they recognize, target, and kill the patient's own tumor cells.

There is hope that research in this area will continue to unlock the mysteries of the immune system and cancer.

Preventing Cancers from Developing

Just as public health experts aim to understand how lifestyle factors, environmental exposures, and genetic elements increase our risks for cancer, several drugs and vaccines are being studied to determine if they can help to reduce the risk of certain cancers.

The goal of chemoprevention is to delay the development of cancer in those at high risk for the disease, not to treat existing cancer. For example, the daily use of some hormonal therapies for up to five years reduces the incidence of breast cancer in high-risk women by about 50 percent. A drug called finasteride, which is in clinical trials, has reduced the number of patients diagnosed with prostate cancer. Aspirin and other members of a class of drugs called non-steroidal anti-inflammatory drugs are also being used to prevent colon cancer.

Chemoprevention drugs may lower the risk of cancer, but they are also known to have side effects. It is important to discuss the risks and benefits of chemoprevention with your doctor.

Vaccines intended to prevent the onset of cancer are called prophylactic vaccines. Prophylactic vaccines are given to healthy individuals before cancer develops. These vaccines are designed to stimulate the immune system to attack viruses that can cause cancer. For example, a virus called Human Papilloma Virus (HPV) is associated with an increased risk of cervical cancer. Based on this finding, two HPV vaccines (Gardasil™ and Cervarix™) have been approved by the FDA to protect young people against HPV, and thus prevent cervical cancer.

Genetic Counseling and Testing

Personalized treatment can also include genetic counseling. Genetic counselors are health care professionals who work with people with a high personal risk of developing cancer. Genetic counselors help to educate patients and families about their hereditary risk and help to create an individualized plan to manage risk that can include genetic testing or ongoing screening.

Genetic testing can screen for the presence of genes found to be linked with cancer, such as BRCA1 and BRCA2 for breast cancer and MSI for colon cancer. These genetic screening methods are used with patients known to be at risk of developing a hereditary cancer, such as someone with

- a family history of cancer (three or more members on the same side of the family with the same or related cancer);
- two or more relatives who were diagnosed with cancer at an early age;
- two or more cancers occurring at different sites in the same relative.

Before undergoing genetic screening, it is important to understand the testing method that is used and its limitations. Genetic screening can relieve anxiety and provide information that allows early medical intervention. For example, women with BRCA1 or BRCA2 mutations who are at high risk for breast cancer may use chemo-preventive medications or opt to undergo prophylactic mastectomy. On the other hand, genetic testing can cause fear or depression or provide a false sense of security if the test is negative.

Although it is becoming more available, genetic counseling is not always covered by insurance or Medicare because its impact is still being studied. As genetic testing improves and more treatments are developed, genetic counseling is likely to become more available and more useful.

Improved Screening for Cancer

Ultimately, even before the best new treatments can be administered, it is most important to identify and diagnose cancers as early and as accurately as possible. When cancer is diagnosed early, patients are much more likely to be cured of the disease. Screening for breast cancer using annual mammograms, for colorectal cancer using colonoscopies, for prostate cancer by measuring PSA levels (until a better test is found), and for cervical cancer using Pap smears are routinely used to look for abnormalities that suggest cancer, and have saved thousands of lives.

New imaging techniques to find cancer early are a high priority for cancer researchers. For example, recent reports indicate that the spiral CT scan (or helical CT scan) is better than the standard chest X-ray in saving lives from lung cancer in current or former heavy smokers.

Personalized Medicine

In the future, oncologists hope that they will be able to identify the best treatment for you, personally, just by studying a tissue sample and cataloging your genetic makeup.

Cancer research focused on figuring out how the genes and proteins in cancer cells are different from those of normal cells will help. The emerging fields of research, called *genomics* and *proteomics* respectively, have played an important role in understanding genetics, moving us closer to more personalized approaches to treatment.

- Genomics is the study of a person's entire genetic makeup, including genes and their functions. It includes classifying an individual's genes then understanding interactions among genes and with the person's environment. Genomics provides information on genetic variations and the level of gene expression within an individual. This can be compared with information known about different cancers and how they function.

- Proteomics is the field of study that seeks to understand the proteins expressed in cells. Proteomics seeks to understand the relationship between a protein's composition, structure, and function as it relates to biological activities including health and disease states.

Biomarkers and Tissue-Sample Research

As more is learned about targets in cancer cells, doctors will use this information to design a treatment plan unique to each particular patient and capable of identifying the risk of cancer recurrence. For example, elevated levels of a protein called cancer antigen-125 (CA125) may help to identify patients with ovarian cancer.

These proteins and other cell elements serve as biomarkers that play an important role in cancer screening. Biomarkers also serve to indicate whether or not an individual will respond to a specific treatment. Scientists have identified over 1,000 potential biomarkers that are being tested to determine whether they are robust enough for use in clinical practice. Scientists are hopeful that this information can lead to tailored cancer prevention for particular patients, and several studies are underway.

People who have cancer are being asked if they will allow their blood samples and/or tumor tissue samples to be stored and studied. By studying the blood and tumor tissue at the cell's molecular level, scientists can do more to identify clues about how a tumor tissue grows, multiplies, and spreads, and look deeper at cell functions, signals, genetic factors, and proteins. Blood- and tissue-sample research is the key to developing better cancer drugs that target cell functions in very specific ways.

Your Role in the Future of Cancer Research

The future of cancer care relies on the willingness of people with cancer to help expand our knowledge of the disease and how to treat it. By learning about the latest treatment advances, by participating in a clinical trial for a new therapy, or by donating your blood or tissue sample to be studied, you can play a valuable role in improving the way cancer is prevented, detected, and treated.

Patient Action Plan

- **Be aware that therapies and treatments are being developed all the time.**
  Search on the NCI's Web site (www.cancer.gov) for "targeted treatments" to see what's new.
- **Become your own "cancer researcher."**
  Stay informed about new developments in personalized treatment.
- **Don't allow yourself to be overwhelmed.**
  There are many new, developing frontiers. Asking questions is the best way to navigate your choices.
- **Consider research participation.**
  You can donate blood or tissue samples or participate in a clinical trial to contribute to the science of improving cancer treatment for future generations.

Chapter 7

Clinical Trials

It's a big decision and it's not for everyone, but I'm really glad I made it. That's why I'm here today.

COLORECTAL CANCER SURVIVOR,
National Institutes of Health clinical trials participant

bEFORE OR DURING the course of your treatment, your doctor may mention, or you may read about, a clinical trial for a new cancer drug that looks promising for your type of cancer. It is worth considering participation in a clinical trial when there is some reason to believe that a treatment under investigation could be a good option for you.

Before giving your consent to participate in a clinical trial, or before you choose any treatment option, you should learn as much as possible about what each treatment is, how it was developed, and what its known risks and benefits are. Ask questions until you're sure that you can make the best decision possible regarding your treatment possibilities.

People participating in clinical trials might be the first to benefit from a new treatment—but 85 percent of cancer patients aren't even aware that clinical trials are a treatment option for them. The majority of studies in cancer are done in clinical trials conducted by the National Cancer Institute (NCI), cancer centers, and the pharmaceutical industry.

How New Cancer Treatments Are Developed and Tested

Before cancer treatments become available to the general public, clinical research studies must show that the treatment is both safe and effective. The first step in this process occurs through basic research in the laboratory with preclinical testing in cells, tissues, and animals. Results from laboratory testing must demonstrate that the new intervention might be effective against cancer before the treatment can be studied in people. The next step involves human research studies, which are commonly referred to as clinical trials.

What Are Clinical Trials?

Clinical trials test new treatments; seek improvements to current treatments; or are aimed at side effects, screening, or preventing cancer recurrence. Clinical trial participants make an important contribution to the future of cancer care.

All new treatments tested in a clinical trial must successfully complete each of three phases of trials before the U.S. Food and Drug Administration (FDA) approves them for general use.

- *Phase I* trials help researchers determine the safety and side effects of the treatment and the most effective way to give the new treatment to patients (by mouth, injection, or IV drip, for instance) and dose. Only a few people participate in this stage of the clinical trial process.
- *Phase II* trials evaluate whether the new treatment actually has a positive effect against a particular type of cancer. If at least 20 percent of participants respond well to the treatment, the new therapy undergoes further evaluation.
- *Phase III* trials compare the new treatment to the most effective existing treatment for a particular type of cancer. If eligible, many people—hundreds or even thousands—can participate. Phase III trials can involve adding a new drug to an already-proven combination of drugs to see if the combination is more effective. It's important to know that, in general, every participant in a Phase III trial receives either the current standard treatment *or* the new treatment. People who are eligible for a clinical trial and choose to participate are informed of the possible risks and benefits and are protected through laws that value a participant's right to drop out of the trial at any time.

> **Research Goals in Clinical Trials**
>
> *Phase I*: Is the drug safe?
> *Phase II*: Does the drug work?
> *Phase III*: How does the drug compare to the best standard of care?

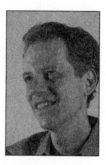

I chose to participate in a clinical trial because I wanted to be as aggressive as possible with my treatment. I also know that these trials are an important part in helping us to learn more about lung cancer and help bring us closer to a cure.

JERRY,
lung cancer survivor

Types of Clinical Trials

Source: National Cancer Institute

- Prevention trials test new approaches, such as medications, vitamins, or other supplements, that doctors believe might lower the risk of developing a certain type of cancer. Most prevention trials are conducted with healthy people who haven't had cancer. Some trials are conducted with people who have had cancer and want to prevent recurrence (return of cancer) or reduce the chance of developing a new type of cancer.
- Screening trials study ways to detect cancer earlier. These trials involve people who do not have any symptoms of cancer.
- Diagnostic trials study tests or procedures that could be used to identify cancer more accurately, and they usually include people who have signs or symptoms of cancer.
- Treatment trials are conducted with people who have cancer. They are designed to answer specific questions about, and evaluate the effectiveness of, a new treatment or a new way to use a standard treatment. These trials test many types of treatments, such as new drugs, vaccines, new approaches to surgery or radiation therapy, or new combinations of treatments.
- Quality-of-life trials (also called supportive care) explore ways to improve the comfort and quality of life of cancer patients and cancer survivors. These trials might study ways to help

people who are experiencing nausea, vomiting, sleep disorders, depression, or other effects from cancer or its treatment.

- Genetic studies are sometimes part of another cancer clinical trial. These trials focus on cellular functions and how genetics can affect detection, diagnosis, or response to cancer treatment.
- Population- and family-based genetic research studies differ from traditional cancer clinical trials. In these studies, researchers look at tissue or blood samples, generally from families or large groups of people, to find genetic changes that are associated with cancer. People who participate in genetic studies might or might not have cancer, depending on the study. The goal of these studies is to help understand the role of genes in the development of cancer.

> **Find a Clinical Trial**
>
> The National Cancer Institute: http://clinicaltrials.gov
> The National Cancer Institute's Cancer Trials Support Unit:
>   www.ctsu.org
> Coalition of National Cancer Cooperative Groups' Trial Check:
>   www.trialcheck.org/services
> Cancer Support Community's Emerging Med Service: 800-814-
>   8927

How Does a Drug Gain FDA Approval?

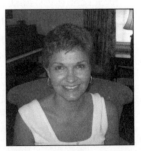

I was the last person chosen for (a) Phase I/II trial of PR1 Peptide vaccine. The support I received (at CSC) helped me to grow spiritually throughout that ordeal. I now go to my local oncologist monthly for CBCs. If my counts are good, I run out the door for another month. There are no promises, projections, or probabilities offered for the duration of my remission. The drug I received is too new for that. I'm learning to live one day at a time....I try to make the best of that, make reasonable plans for the future, and then turn it over to God.

KIMBERLY HENRY,
Cancer Support Community, East Tennessee

If the data obtained from a completed Phase III trial shows that a new treatment is safe and effective at saving or extending the lives of patients, the sponsor of the trial can then submit an application to the FDA for approval of the treatment. Scientists at the FDA analyze the data brought to them to ensure that safety and efficacy have been established. After extensive review, if the FDA is satisfied with the results, approval is granted and the drug then becomes available on the market.

For a very small percentage of treatments in clinical trials, the FDA offers "expanded-access" programs to make promising new treatments available to the public outside of the traditional clinical trial setting. Expanded access programs are mostly for people with serious or life-threatening illnesses and without other treatment options, even before these drugs are formally approved by the FDA for the public's use.

Informed Consent

Before you join a clinical trial, a health care professional will explain the purpose of the trial and what you'll be asked to do. You can ask questions about the trial and will be given a detailed consent form to read and sign. The informed consent process begins with the initial explanation from your doctor, the document you sign to start treatment, and then ongoing information provided to you throughout the course of your treatment. The consent form must include the following information:

- a statement that explains the purposes of the research, the expected time frame of participation, a description of the procedures that are experimental, and how the clinical trial will be conducted;
- any likely side effects from the treatment;
- an explanation of alternative treatment options, if any exist;
- a statement describing the confidentiality of your medical records;
- for trials involving more than minimal risk, an explanation of potential injuries and compensation—if any—available due to injury, treatments available if injury occurs, and resources for further information;
- an explanation of whom to contact for answers to questions about the research and participants' rights;

- a statement that participation is voluntary, that refusal to participate will not have penalties or loss of benefits; and that you may discontinue participation at any time without penalty.

Here are some important questions you should ask your doctor before choosing to participate in a clinical trial (some of these questions will be answered in the informed consent document).

- What is the purpose of the study?
- Why would it be important as a treatment option for me?
- What kinds of tests and treatments are done as part of the study?
- What are my potential benefits and risks compared to other treatment options?
- What are the eligibility requirements?
- How could the clinical trial affect my daily life?
- What will happen to my cancer with or without this new treatment?
- What are other treatment choices?
- How long will the study last?
- Where will I have to go for treatment?
- Will my insurance company, Medicare, Medicaid, or the funder of the study cover the costs? Will there be out-of-pocket costs for me?
- Who will help me answer coverage questions?
- What type of long-term and follow-up care is part of the study?

Benefits and Risks to Participation

Below are the benefits of participating in a clinical trial, according to the NCI.

- Participants have access to promising new treatments that are not available outside the clinical trial setting.
- The approach being studied might be more effective than the standard approach.
- Participants receive regular and careful medical attention from a research team that includes doctors and other health professionals.

- Participants might be the first to benefit from the new method under study.
- Results from the study will help others in the future.

Below are the risks of participating in a clinical trial.

- New drugs or procedures under study are not always better than the standard care to which they are being compared.
- New treatments can have side effects or risks that doctors don't expect or that are worse than those resulting from standard care.
- Participants in randomized trials won't be able to choose the approach they receive.
- Health insurance and managed care providers might not cover all patient care costs, including out-of-pocket costs (e.g., child care, transportation) in a study.
- Participants might be required to make more visits to the doctor than they would if they were not in the clinical trial.

Source: National Cancer Institute

Are You Protected During a Clinical Trial?

Research with humans is conducted according to strict scientific and ethical principles. Every clinical trial has a protocol or action plan that serves as a "recipe" for conducting the trial. The plan describes what will be done in the study, how it will be conducted, and why each part of the study is necessary. The same protocol is used by every doctor or research center taking part in the trial.

All clinical trials that are federally funded or that evaluate a new drug or medical device subject to FDA regulation must be reviewed and approved by an Institutional Review Board (IRB). An IRB, which includes doctors, researchers, community leaders, and other members of the community, reviews the protocol initially and throughout the clinical trial to make sure the study is conducted fairly and that participants aren't likely to be harmed. After review, the IRB can recommend changes or stop a clinical trial if the researcher isn't following the protocol or if the trial appears to be causing unexpected harm to the participants. An

IRB can also stop a clinical trial early if there's clear evidence that the new intervention is effective and should be widely available.

Clinical trials supported by the National Institutes of Health require data and safety monitoring. Some clinical trials, especially Phase III clinical trials, use a Data and Safety Monitoring Board (DSMB). A DSMB is an independent committee made up of statisticians, physicians, and patient advocates. The DSMB ensures that the risks of participation are as small as possible, makes sure the data are complete, and stops a trial if safety concerns arise or when the trial's objectives have been met.

Source: National Cancer Institute

Who Pays for Clinical Trials?

Health insurance and managed care providers might not cover the patient care costs associated with a clinical trial. Coverage varies by health plan and by study. Some health plans do not cover clinical trials if they consider the approach being studied "experimental" or "investigational." In many cases, it helps to have someone from the research team talk about coverage with representatives of the health plan.

More information about insurance coverage can be found on the NCI's *Clinical Trials and Insurance Coverage: A Resource Guide* Web page (www.cancer.gov/clinicaltrials/learning/insurance-coverage). The Cancer Support Community's (CSC's) publication, *Frankly Speaking about Cancer: Coping with the Cost of Care*, also covers some of these issues (go to www.cancersupportcommunity.org to order free materials).

Many states have passed legislation or developed policies requiring health plans to cover the costs of certain clinical trials. For more information, visit the NCI's Web site at: www.cancer.gov/clinicaltrials/developments/laws-about-clinical-trial-costs.

Federal programs that help pay the costs of care in a clinical trial include those listed below.

- Medicare reimburses patient care costs for beneficiaries who participate in clinical trials designed to diagnose or treat cancer. Information about Medicare coverage of clinical trials is available at www.medicare.gov, or by calling Medicare's toll-free number for beneficiaries at 800-MEDICARE (800-633-4227). The toll-free number for the hearing impaired is 877-486-2048. Also, the NCI fact sheet, *More Choices in Cancer Care: Information for Beneficiaries on Medicare Coverage of Cancer Clinical Trials,* is available at: www.cancer.gov/cancertopics/factsheet/support/medicare.

- Beneficiaries of TRICARE, the Department of Defense's health program, can be reimbursed for the medical costs of participation in NCI-sponsored Phase II and Phase III cancer prevention (including screening and early detection) and treatment trials. Additional information is available in the NCI fact sheet, *TRICARE Beneficiaries Can Enter Clinical Trials for Cancer Prevention and Treatment Through a Department of Defense and National Cancer Institute Agreement.* This fact sheet can be found at: www.cancer.gov/cancertopics/factsheet/NCI/TRICARE.
- The Department of Veterans Affairs (VA) allows eligible veterans to participate in NCI-sponsored prevention, diagnosis, and treatment studies nationwide. All phases and types of NCI-sponsored trials are included. The NCI fact sheet, *The NCI/VA Agreement on Clinical Trials: Questions and Answers,* has more information. It's available at: http://previewqa.cancer.gov/cancertopics/factsheet/NCI/Fs1_17.pdf.

Source: National Cancer Institute

The Long-Term Impact of Research on Patients

Information gathered from research studies tells doctors which treatments, including dosages, schedules, and combinations, work or don't work in patients. Results from clinical trials continue to determine the *standard of care,* the best treatment approach for a patient's type and stage of cancer. Standard of care treatments typically demonstrate a proven benefit through an increase in survival, decrease in the size of the tumor or extensiveness of the disease, or improved quality of life through a reduction in side effects.

Many types of cancer are being treated as a chronic disease to be controlled over time. Even those cancers diagnosed in later stages might be managed over the course of several years. Therefore, oncologists and patients are shifting their treatment strategies to consider long-term health issues. This shift is directed toward the goal of enabling a person with cancer to function at his or her maximum level for as long as possible.

Researchers will continue to study new treatments until every type of cancer can be prevented or cured.

Patient Action Plan

- **Seek a second opinion at a cancer center that participates actively in cancer clinical trials.**
  If you want to consider a clinical trial, discuss your options with an oncologist at a large cancer center that actively participates in cancer research.
- **Partner with your physician.**
  Before deciding to enroll in a clinical trial, schedule a meeting with your oncologist. Bring a family member or friend to help you address your questions and concerns.
- **Find support.**
  Talk with others who have experience with a clinical trial. Your health care team or organizations such as the Cancer Support Community will help connect you with others who can share their experiences.
- **Educate yourself.**
  There are organizations that provide up-to-date information about what's being studied and whether a cancer clinical trial is right for you.

Chapter 8

Considering Another Approach:
Complementary and Alternative Medicine

Rarely in life does one have the opportunity to receive for themselves the benefits of their gifts. For years I have shared inspired harp music with patients and families in cancer, hospice, and grief communities around the country, offering a sense of peace, hope, and comfort as they journey from day to day. Now, I am one of those patients being comforted by that same music, expressed from the deepest part of my soul.

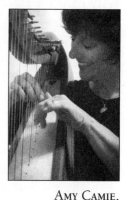

AMY CAMIE,
community member, Cancer Support Community,
Greater St. Louis

WHEN YOU'RE MOTIVATED by the desire to recover and get relief from cancer symptoms and side effects, you might consider treatments that your doctor doesn't mention, such as acupuncture or dietary supplements. The National Center for Complementary and Alternative Medicine (NCCAM), part of the National Institutes of Health (NIH), defines these types of treatments as Complementary and Alternative Medicines (also known as "CAM"). They are a "group of diverse medical and health care systems, practices, and products that are not considered to be a standard part of conventional medicine." Other examples of CAM treatments include meditation, yoga, and other relaxation techniques; chiropractic services; biofeedback or energy techniques; music and art therapy; and dietary or herbal products.

In essence, CAM practices have become attractive to more and more people annually. The 2007 National Health Interview Survey (NHIS) showed that about 40 percent of cancer patients in the United States use some form of CAM. The most popular CAM therapies among cancer survivors were herbal and other natural products (20 percent), deep breathing (14 percent), and meditation (9 percent). This chapter will help you navigate the various CAM treatments available so that you and your doctor can make informed decisions about what's right for you.

Why People Use CAM

Some CAM therapies have been scientifically studied to see whether they are effective. Many others haven't been studied, so it is still unknown whether they're safe or effective—or even how they work. As of now, no scientific studies have shown that complementary or alternative therapy alone can cure disease, and most of these treatments are not covered by insurance, but CAM can

- relieve cancer symptoms and the side effects of treatment;
- control pain and improve comfort;
- relieve stress and anxiety;
- enhance physical, emotional, and spiritual well-being;
- improve quality of life.

Alternative medicines are used to replace conventional therapies. If someone opts to use herbal supplements to treat cancer instead of chemotherapy or radiation, he or she would be using an alternative treatment. Alternative treatments may seem to offer hope when conventional treatments fail, but they're often unproven and can even be dangerous. If using an alternative treatment delays the use of a conventional treatment, then it can radically diminish the likelihood of remission and cure.

As a complement to conventional treatments, CAM can be a useful tool. If you do choose to pursue CAM, make sure you learn as much as possible about your choice—and, as always, be sure to include your doctor and caregiver in your decision-making process.

CAM CHOICE GUIDELINES
Tell your doctor about your CAM use.
Carefully select the CAM practitioner to ensure quality and professionalism.
Know that products called "natural" are not necessarily safe.
Use information only from trusted resources, such as the National Center for Complementary and Alternative Medicine (http://nccam.nih.gov/).
Feel free to tell friends and family offering advice that you, your doctor, and your caregiver have come up with a CAM game plan with which you are comfortable, but you appreciate their concern for you.

There are five major categories of CAM: alternative medical systems; mind-body interventions; biologically based therapies; manipulative and body-based systems; and energy therapies. Let's explore each one in greater detail.

Alternative Medical Systems: Achieving Mind-Body Harmony

Alternative medical systems include ayurveda, homeopathy, naturopathy, and traditional Chinese medicine. All of these are complete systems of theory and practice, and some have been used for centuries. A central theme to these systems is the goal of achieving harmony of mind and body. However, the basic assumptions and understandings of how disease unfolds in these systems don't fit with current Western scientific understanding, which makes it more challenging to use these systems in conjunction with conventional medicine. However, you might still find elements in each system that are useful to you for CAM practices, such as mind-centering, prayer, exercise, and relaxation.

Ayurvedic Medicine

Ayurvedic medicine has been practiced primarily in the Indian subcontinent for 5,000 years. People are classified into one of three body types that determine which herbal remedies and dietary regimens they should use. In ayurveda, the key to preventing and treating disease is a balanced consciousness; yoga and meditation are primary techniques used to maintain and promote that balance.

Homeopathic Medicine

Homeopathic medicine originated in Germany in the eighteenth century based on the principle that "like cures like." Small, highly diluted amounts of medicinal substances derived from plants, minerals, and animals are used to treat symptoms. In higher doses, these substances would actually cause symptoms. For instance, a poison ivy rash is treated by applying a solution of highly diluted poison ivy oil to the rash.

Clinical trials and systemic reviews have not found homeopathy to be a proven treatment for any medical condition. Some research indicates that homeopathy works due to the placebo effect: If the patient believes it will work, it might help him or her, but relying on this type of treatment on its own for any cancer could have negative consequences.

Naturopathic Medicine

Naturopathic medicine includes many approaches to healing, including: dietary modifications, massage, exercise, stress reduction, acupuncture, and conventional medicine. Practitioners believe that if a healthy internal environment exists, the body will heal itself.

There is no scientific evidence that naturopathic medicine cures cancer or any other disease. Most of these methods won't harm you, but some herbal preparations can be toxic; for instance, fasting, limiting diet, and the use of enemas could be dangerous if used excessively. Relying on naturopathic medicine as your sole treatment against cancer could also have negative consequences. On the other hand, massage, exercise, and stress-reduction techniques are all excellent for overall health, and when used in conjunction with conventional treatment (and planned between you and your doctor), these techniques can be highly beneficial.

Traditional Chinese Medicine

Traditional Chinese medicine (TCM) views the body as an ecosystem that needs to stay in balance; opposing forces in the system can cause imbalance, disrupt the flow of energy (or Chi), and produce illness.

The goal of TCM is to maintain and promote balance within the body to restore positive energy flow. Herbal remedies, acupuncture, massage, and meditative physical exercise are all used as treatment. While the anti-cancer effects of TCM might be limited, many practices, such as acupuncture, have been shown to reduce side effects such as nausea and stress caused by cancer treatment. Acupuncture has also been shown to be effective when combined with drugs for controlling post-operative pain in some patients.

More research is needed to assess the effectiveness of herbal remedies and other TCM practices.

Mind-Body Interventions

Mind-body interventions are the second category in the five major types of CAM. Different techniques are used to influence the mind's ability to affect bodily function and systems. Mind-body interventions with which you may be familiar include prayer; meditation; guided imagery; and art, music, or dance therapy.

Prayer for health reasons, also called faith healing or spiritual coping, is utilized by many people. People have different ideas about life after death, miracles, and other religious beliefs. The impact of prayer, spirituality, and religion on the well-being of cancer patients and their loved ones is very interesting but is also very unknown.

Meditation relaxes the body and calms the mind, often creating a feeling of well-being. Different types of meditation (Zen, Vipassana, and Transcendental Meditation) can be self-directed or guided. Meditation involves being in a quiet place and focusing on an object of meditation, which could be breath, a mantra, or the physical sensations of slow walking. Although there is no scientific evidence to prove that meditation treats cancer or any other disease, when used regularly, the practice has been shown to have some beneficial physiological and psychological effects. Clinical trials have found meditation useful in reducing anxiety, stress, blood pressure, chronic pain, and insomnia.

Guided imagery practitioners help patients train the mind to produce a physiological or psychological effect using images and symbols. Guided imagery is based on the principle that if you think about calming images and thoughts, your body will feel calm, which is important for your physical well-being.

Biologically Based Therapies

Biologically based therapies use substances that are found in nature, including herbs, certain foods or diets, and vitamins. Examples include dietary supplements, herbal products, and other "natural"—but unproven—therapies. Remember, a "natural" product does NOT necessarily mean a "safe" product! Please be aware that herbal products and vitamins might keep other medicines, such as chemotherapy, from doing what they are supposed to do.

Dietary supplements include vitamins; minerals; herbs or other botanicals; amino acids; and substances such as enzymes, organ tissues, and metabolites. Dietary supplements come in many forms, including extracts, concentrates, tablets, gel capsules, liquids, and powders. They are considered foods, not drugs, so there are no regulations controlling their safety, content, quality, or dose recommendations. Unless they are proven unsafe, the U.S. Food and Drug Administration (FDA) does not require manufacturers to print side effects on the labels of these products or remove them from the market.

Dietary supplements have different active substances, so their effectiveness must be assessed individually. The American Cancer Society (ACS; www.cancer.org) has an extensive listing of dietary supplements on its Web site, and offers guidance through supporters and critics.

Herbal products are used in many different types of natural medicine. In the United States, herbal medicine generally refers to a system of medicine that uses European or North American plants. Ayurvedic medicine uses plants from India, and TCM uses plants from China. Modern herbalists often use plants from many different regions of the world. Because herbs and roots have different active substances, and they are also considered foods, there is also no regulation regarding their safety or efficacy.

Manipulative and Body-Based Systems

Manipulative and body-based systems are practices based on physical manipulation and/or movement of one or more parts of the body. Examples include chiropractic or osteopathic manipulation and massage. There could be great risk associated with these types of therapies if a patient has bone metastases. As with any CAM treatments, you should consult with your physician first before utilizing these therapies.

Chiropractic practices focus on the relationship between bodily structure—primarily that of the spine—and function, and how that relationship affects health. Chiropractors use physical manipulation as an integral treatment tool. There's no scientific evidence that chiropractic treatment cures cancer or any other disease. Although treatment has been shown to help treat lower back pain and other pain, due to muscle or bone problems, and to promote relaxation and stress reduction, complications can occur in a small number of cases.

Osteopathic practice is a form of conventional medicine emphasizing diseases that arise in the musculoskeletal system. It's grounded in a belief that the body's systems work together and that disturbances in one system can affect the functioning of another. Some osteopathic physicians practice a full-body system of hands-on manipulation to alleviate pain, restore function, and promote health and well-being. There is little scientific evidence that osteopathy is effective in treating cancer, or any other condition, except musculoskeletal problems. Some reports suggest that people with bone cancer should not use osteopathy.

Massage is when therapists manipulate and knead muscle and connective tissue to enhance function of those tissues and to promote relaxation and well-being. It can be used to relieve joint pain, reduce stiffness, rehabilitate injured muscles, and reduce pain. Recent studies suggest that massage can lower levels of stress, anxiety, depression, and pain. It can also have effects on fatigue, blood pressure, and quality of sleep. Massage that is conducted by a trained, licensed professional is regarded as safe. In the past, there was concern that people with cancer should not receive massage because tissue manipulation might cause cancer cells to migrate. No evidence has been found, however, to suggest that this will occur.

Energy Therapies

Energy therapies are based on a theory that there are energy fields around the human body. It is believed that by changing the energy fields by manual manipulation, such as QiGong or healing touch, disease can be eliminated. Overall, energy therapies are considered to be questionable as far as treating disease, although many people with cancer relate that they find these practices to be helpful in reducing stress.

Types of Energy Therapies

There are two types of energy therapies.
- Biofield therapies are meant to influence energy fields that theoretically surround and penetrate the body. Examples include QiGong, Reiki, and therapeutic touch.

• Bioelectromagnetic-based therapies involve using
  electromagnetic fields. Examples include pulsed fields,
  magnetic fields, or alternating current/direct current fields.

QiGong is a component of TCM that combines movement, meditation, and regulation of breathing to enhance the flow of Chi (an ancient
term referring to "vital energy") in the body; improve blood circulation;
and enhance immune function. There is no scientific evidence showing that QiGong can treat cancer or any other disease; however, it can
enhance peace and well-being. According to limited scientific literature,
QiGong might also reduce chronic pain for a short period of time and
relieve anxiety.

Reiki is a Japanese word representing Universal Life Energy. Reiki is
based on the belief that when spiritual energy is channeled through a
Reiki practitioner, the patient's spirit is healed, which in turn heals the
physical body. No scientific studies show that Reiki is effective for treating
cancer or any other disease. However, it, too, could be useful as a complementary therapy to help reduce stress and improve quality of life.

Therapeutic or healing touch is derived from an ancient technique
called "laying on of hands," based on the premise that it is the healing
force of the therapist that affects the patient's recovery. Healing is promoted when the body's energies are in balance, and, by passing their
hands over the patient, healers can identify energy imbalances. There's
no evidence to support that therapeutic touch (TT) balances or trans-
fers energy, because very few well-designed studies of TT have been
conducted. While one study published in the *Journal of the American
Medical Association* (JAMA, 1998) demonstrated that experienced TT
practitioners were unable to detect the energy fields of the investigator,
TT is taught in many nursing schools and is still widely practiced. Some
patients have found that it helps reduce anxiety and increase feelings
of well-being. Many researchers believe that these results are due to the
placebo effect. Note, however, that there's no consistent training or cer-
tifying organization to ensure the level of practice of the provider.

Electromagnetic fields (EMFs) are "invisible lines of force" that surround all electrical devices. Practitioners claim disease occurs when
electromagnetic frequencies or fields of energy within the body are
"out of balance." They believe electromagnetic imbalances disturb the
body's chemistry. By applying electrical energy from outside the body,

usually with electronic devices, practitioners say they can correct these imbalances. However, there's no scientific evidence that electromagnetic therapy is effective in diagnosing or treating cancer or any other disease; many of the alternative electronic devices promoted to cure disease have not been scientifically proven to be effective.

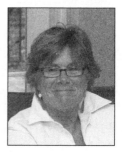

Exercise really helps. I originally felt very uncomfortable after my reconstruction—I lost arm movement after my latissimus dorsi surgery. Physical therapy, swimming, and yoga helped me feel so much better and re-gain movement.

Liz,
breast cancer survivor

Eastern Exercises

Yoga is a form of exercise, usually anaerobic, that involves a sequence of postures and breathing activities. It can relieve some symptoms associated with cancer and other chronic diseases. A system of personal development from the Hindu tradition, it combines dietary guidelines, physical exercise, and meditation to create "prana," or vital energy. Research has found yoga to be beneficial to control bodily functions like blood pressure, heart rate, respiration, and metabolism. It can lead to improved physical fitness and lower levels of stress.

T'ai chi is an ancient Chinese martial art form. It's a mind-body system that uses movement, meditation, and breathing to improve health and well-being. Research has shown that T'ai chi is useful for improving posture, balance, muscle mass and tone, flexibility, stamina, and strength in older adults. T'ai chi is also an effective method for reducing stress.

The Controversy over Alternative Diets

Diet and vitamin cancer "cures" have not been found to be scientifically effective as cancer treatments. Still, nutrition during and after cancer treatment is an important subject for people with cancer, as well as their loved ones (see Chapter 15).

It's hard to make sense of all the available information related to anti-cancer diets, although there are several popular approaches worthy of a closer look. Please remember that none of these approaches has been scientifically proven to prevent or eliminate cancer. Still, you might find that a registered dietician can be helpful in improving your nutritional practices during cancer treatment and beyond. There are registered dieticians certified in oncology who can provide personalized support (American Dietetic Association, or ADA: www.oncologynutrition.org/members/locator).

Macrobiotic diet: A vegetarian diet consisting predominantly of whole grains and cereals (50–60 percent), cooked vegetables and organic fruits (20–25 percent), and soups made with vegetables, seaweed, grains, beans, and miso (5–10 percent). Proponents believe that such a diet can prevent and cure disease, including cancer, and enhance feelings of well-being, although there have been no clinical trials to show that a macrobiotic diet can indeed prevent or cure cancer. Earlier forms of the diet, which involved restricting the diet to brown rice and water, were associated with severe nutritional deficiencies.

Fasting: Fasting entails not eating any food and drinking only water or fruit juice for two to five days or sometimes longer. Practitioners believe that fasting cleanses the body of toxins, but this belief is not supported by scientific research. The body cannot distinguish between fasting and starvation, and cancer studies suggest fasting might actually promote tumor growth.

No matter what, it is best to focus on eating a healthful diet that includes whole grains, fruits, vegetables, fewer foods with saturated fats, and fewer processed foods. Maintaining a healthy weight is always beneficial, in terms of overall well-being and even in terms of reducing the chance that cancer will return after treatment is complete.

What You Should Know If You Use CAM

- **Some CAM therapies are safe, but others are not.**
  Tell your doctor which CAM practices you are using or would like to use. The fact that a product is called "natural" does not necessarily mean it is "safe." For example, the safety of dietary supplements and herbs depends on the ingredients in the product, where those ingredients are from, and whether they have been contaminated during manufacturing. Herbs and supplements can interact with other medications or prevent

them from working. For this and other reasons, it is critical to talk to your doctor about CAM therapies. He or she can help you to understand the risks and benefits of a therapy. Be aware that each person reacts differently to treatments, and all medical therapies can have risks.

- **It's important to be an informed consumer.**
  Learn as much as you can about therapies you are thinking of trying. Understanding the risks, potential benefits, and evidence of effectiveness for CAM therapies is vital to your safety. For many CAM therapies, few scientific studies of their effectiveness have been conducted. However, the National Center for Complementary and Alternative Medicine (NCCAM) is a good source for learning about existing studies (see Appendix for more detailed resource information). You can also use the Internet to search PubMed, a database of medical literature, which has a listing of brief summaries of CAM studies, developed by NCCAM and the National Library of Medicine. In some cases, you can click on a link to view or purchase the full articles. Another database, International Bibliographic Information on Dietary Supplements, is useful for finding scientific literature about dietary supplements.

- **Information from Web sites should be viewed with a critical eye.**
  The Internet is a wonderful resource that allows you to obtain volumes of information with the click of a mouse, but not all of that information is accurate. For this reason, evaluate Web sites with a critical eye. Look for sites that have been established by government agencies, universities, or reputable medical or health-related associations. Educational sites are more credible than those designed to sell a product. Information on the Web sites should include clear references from scientific journals; personal stories are not adequate to back up statements. The information should also be current and recently updated. Be skeptical of sites that ask you for money or make claims that sound "too good to be true."

- **The federal government is a good resource for information about therapies you are considering.**
  If you are considering a therapy, check with the FDA's Web site, www.fda.gov, to see if it has information about that

therapy. The FDA's Center for Food Safety and Applied Nutrition Web site has information about dietary supplements at www.fda.gov/Food/DietarySupplements. You can also visit the FDA's Web site on recalls and safety alerts at www.fda.gov/Safety/Recalls/default.htm. The Web site of the Federal Trade Commission, www.ftc.gov, offers information about consumer alerts for fraudulent therapies. Visit the NCCAM Web site, http://nccam.nih.gov, to see if it has information on the therapy.

- **You can always check a CAM practitioner's credentials.** Licensed and credentialed practitioners can provide higher quality care than unlicensed ones. Credentials don't ensure that a practitioner is competent, but they show that he or she has met certain standards to treat patients. The training, skill, and experience of the practitioner affect safety, so ask your physician or someone you believe is knowledgeable regarding CAM for recommendations. Hospitals and medical schools sometimes keep lists of area CAM practitioners, and some may have a CAM center or CAM practitioners on staff. Contact a professional organization for the type of practitioner you're seeking. Finally, many states have regulatory agencies or licensing boards that can tell you about practitioners in your area.

Quackwatch and Other Watchdog Groups

Quackwatch, Inc. is one example of a nonprofit organization that aims to identify health-related frauds, myths, fads, and fallacies. This group primarily tries to expose quackery or "pretenders in medical skill, those who talk pretentiously without sound knowledge of the subject discussed." Quackwatch is useful for gaining background information on a questionable CAM topic or when information is difficult or impossible to find elsewhere. The services mentioned above can be found on www.quackwatch.org.

Patient Action Plan

This helpful "to-do" list is adapted from suggestions on the American Cancer Society's Web site and NCCAM:

- **Gather as much information as possible on your own.**
  Seek information from reputable, credible sources on the potential benefits and risks of the CAM practice you are considering.
- **Ask your oncologist questions about the CAM practice you are considering.**
  Listen to what he or she says about it; try to understand that perspective. If the CAM treatment will cause problems with your cancer treatment or is considered to be fraudulent by an oncologist, discuss safer alternatives together.
- **Don't delay or forego conventional cancer treatment.**
  If you consider stopping or not taking conventional treatment, please discuss this decision with your doctor. Remember that you may be giving up the only proven treatment.
- **If you are taking dietary supplements, make a complete list of what you are taking and show your oncologist.**
  Many supplements can interact in potentially harmful ways with cancer treatment. Report any changes to your health care team.
- **Choose a practitioner based on his or her experience and treatment history.**
  This is especially important if you seek care from an acupuncturist or chiropractor, for example.
- **Tell all of your health practitioners about the full picture of what you do to manage your health.**
  This proactive step will help ensure coordination and safe care.

Chapter 9

Managing Symptoms and Side Effects

When it comes to side effects, it's extremely important to relay everything you're experiencing to your doctor. There may be a solution or it may lend critical information for your care.

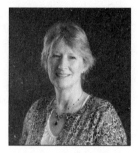

GINNY,
breast cancer survivor

eVERY PERSON'S EXPERIENCE with cancer treatment is unique. You might not experience every possible side effect, but being aware of what might happen can help reassure you that certain side effects are anticipated, and as a result, help you feel prepared.

The most important thing you can do is to be a proactive participant in your own disease management.

Being informed about side effects enables you and your doctor to prevent or proactively manage problems before they disrupt your treatment or decrease your quality of life. Being proactive also means reporting any symptoms or side effects you experience to your health care team immediately, so you can work together to control them.

"Is It the Cancer . . . or Something Else?"

Many cancer patients have shared that, ever since their diagnosis, they've become very conscious of their bodies. Some worry that they may stress too much about "every ache and pain" and can't tell when something is really wrong. Do you often wonder if an ache or other symptom is a sign of cancer progressing? It's important that you learn to read your physical signs, keep track of symptoms and side effects, and communicate with your health care team regularly.

No question is ever too insignificant to ask. More often than not, the signs and symptoms you're experiencing are temporary and related to the treatment you are receiving. If you experience a side effect from therapy, it doesn't mean that something is wrong, that the drugs you're taking aren't destroying cancer cells, or that the cancer has necessarily progressed. However, it does mean that you must be vigilant and maintain open communication with your team so that you can keep your treatment on track and commit to feeling as good as possible.

Be proactive in asserting what you need to prevent or control side effects. Be clear with your health care team about how particular symptoms are impacting your day-to-day life.

The easiest way to understand what you're experiencing is to be well informed. By knowing what potential side effects can occur, you can alert your doctor or nurse of their occurrence before they become severe—and before you get yourself in a quandary over whether or not these concerns are related to the treatment or to the cancer itself.

Remember, this is when being an empowered patient becomes so important.

No one ever said that just because you have cancer you have to suffer. Thanks to phenomenal advances in supportive treatments, cancer therapy doesn't have to be as miserable as you might think. You can do it: Be informed—take action!

Staying on Schedule

It's important that your treatment remains on schedule. After all, you want to get through your treatment quickly and successfully, right? Having to postpone your treatment due to side effects can leave you feeling disappointed, anxious, and fearful. This is why managing side effects improves the way you feel during treatment; it could also make a difference in the outcome of your treatment.

Delays in treatment are certainly emotionally troubling. In a study of 500 chemotherapy patients, 37 percent of those who experienced a delay due to a low white cell count said they found the delay to be "extremely" or "somewhat" stressful. Worse, 31 percent of those patients who had to delay treatment said they felt emotionally troubled enough to want to quit their treatment at some point.

In this guidebook, we provide some suggestions for managing the most common side effects experienced by cancer patients. Additional information about side effect management can be found in the Cancer Support Community's (CSC's) free booklet, *Frankly Speaking About Cancer Treatments: Take Control of Side Effects with Medicine, Mind and Body*; online at www.cancersupportcommunity.org; or through the National Cancer Institute's (NCI's) Web site (www.cancer.gov).

> *It can get harsh with treatment; she gets really tired and sluggish— and it gets hard to plan for things. So it's the little things, like laying on the couch and just hanging out with a movie, that helps us relax.*

> MICHAEL,
> caregiver

Fatigue

Nearly all people who are treated for cancer experience cancer-related fatigue. It is the most frequently registered complaint of patients with cancer and, often, the most distressing.

The National Comprehensive Cancer Network (NCCN) defines fatigue as a distressing, persistent sense of tiredness or exhaustion related to cancer or cancer treatment that is not proportional to recent activity and interferes with normal functioning. The NCCN Guidelines recommend that you be assessed for the effects of fatigue as often as is needed.

Did You Know...

- Too much rest, as well as too little rest, contributes to increased feelings of fatigue?
- Too little activity, as well as too much activity, can cause feelings of fatigue?
- Everyday energy expenditure is the most potent regulator of the body's energy systems? (With energy, it's a "use it or lose it" proposition.)

- Feeling fatigued can make you feel more distressed about other symptoms or concerns?
- How you feel about other symptoms or concerns can lead to feelings of fatigue?

How Much Fatigue Will I Experience—and For How Long?

It's difficult to predict how fatigued you will feel, because it tends to be different from person to person. Some therapies, such as bone marrow or stem cell transplants, some biotherapies, and certain radiotherapies, cause more fatigue than others. In most cases, you'll gradually begin to feel less fatigued when your treatment ends.

What Can I Do to Avoid the Effects of Fatigue?

Part of managing fatigue is discovering the causes and putting a plan of action into place to deal with the fatigue during treatment. Your health care team will want to know

- if you're having problems with pain or difficulty sleeping;
- whether you're experiencing emotional distress or depression;
- what your activity levels have been;
- how well you're eating and drinking;
- whether you're anemic or at risk for anemia (low red blood cells);
- what other illnesses you might have or medications you're taking.

It's important to be honest about the medications you're taking (prescribed, herbals, vitamins, and other over-the-counter medicines). Some medicines and combinations of medications can contribute to fatigue, and it's possible to adjust medicine regimens to avoid making the fatigue worse.

Fatigue is an unwelcome, but expected, result of cancer treatment. Feeling fatigued isn't itself an indication that your cancer is worse. Discuss fatigue regularly with your health care team, so that strategies can be put in place to help you.

Conserve Your Energy!

There are several easy ways to help you conserve energy and prevent fatigue.

- Delegate tasks to others.
- Nap in the early afternoon—short power-naps, not long enough to interfere with nighttime sleep.
- Avoid caffeine in the evening.
- Schedule activities or structure your routine to accomplish tasks.
- Keep a regular daily routine that is reasonable, considering your abilities.
- Take short walks, or do light exercise, if possible.
- Set realistic goals that you can meet without too much effort.
- Drink water during the day.
- Eat a well-balanced diet with frequent, small meals.
- Learn mind-body techniques to de-stress and relax.

Engage your family and friends to help you accomplish tasks that are important to you, and permit others to relieve you of responsibilities and work that can be completed for you. Near your phone, keep a list of tasks that need to be done. When friends call to ask how they can help, give them a task from your list. You should view this as a good opportunity to take control of your life and the situation.

A Few Words About "Chemo-Brain"

Many people who've gone through cancer treatment say they experience what survivors call "chemo-brain." Symptoms include forgetfulness, lack of concentration, difficulty finding the right word(s), and problems with multitasking. If you feel like you have chemo-brain, talk with your doctor and try some of these helpful tips.

- Simplify your life by doing one thing at a time.
- Carry a personal calendar or notebook to keep notes and make lists.
- Reduce stress and improve focus with relaxation and meditation practices.
- Take classes or do puzzles to "exercise your brain."
- Eat your veggies (studies show that nutrients from vegetables improves brain function).

What About Exercise?

There is a large body of research demonstrating the physical and emotional benefits of exercise for cancer patients. Exercise reduces fatigue, distress, anxiety, and depression; it also helps with weight control, endurance, sexual functioning, and your ability to do the things that are meaningful and important to you. Best of all, exercise can help you feel mentally alert, emotionally calm, and physically energized.

Because cancer treatments can make you feel fatigued, exercise can help you generate more energy and feel physically and emotionally equipped to deal with your illness and life. Although exercise won't make your cancer go away, it's something you can do to feel better, get through treatment more easily, and stay healthy after treatment ends.

You can ask your physician for a referral to a physical therapist or cancer rehabilitation program if you feel this kind of support will help you. If you don't ask, these extended services may not be readily offered. You can also create your own exercise program. CSC affiliates around the country offer gentle exercise programs in yoga, T'ai chi, and others to help patients get started.

Long after treatment is behind you, it's important to be proactive in maintaining your health. Exercise can help you maintain a healthy body weight and reduce your risk for heart disease and diabetes—and perhaps even the risk of a cancer recurrence. It's always one of the most important things you can do for yourself!

Customized Exercise after Cancer

The simple idea behind a customized routine: If it feels good, do it! If it feels bad, adapt it! Start slowly, and be patient. Exercise during cancer treatment is a balance. More isn't always better, but some is important.

Customized exercise is about "reading" your body and changing an exercise movement to fit how you feel on a given day to accommodate any physical or other limitations you may have.

Begin your routine well below what you could do before treatment started, and progress in step-by-step fashion to regain strength. In time, you'll be able to do more exercise with less effort. You *do* want to continue the exercise rather than quit—even when you are not feeling your best or when you are fatigued—because of the many positive benefits mentioned above.

Cancer Transitions: Moving Beyond Treatment™ is a six-week, community-based program for cancer survivors hosted by CSC affiliates and partners. The program was created by CSC in partnership with LIVE**STRONG**. It includes education on medical issues, exercise and nutrition lessons, and emotional support. It is designed to help patients understand and take charge of their lives after cancer.

Customized Exercise Recommendations

Here are some customized exercise recommendations following treatment.

- If you feel sick, exercise only as much or as strenuously as you can. Any exercise is better than none. Start gently, slowly, and for brief periods.
- Be sure to breathe deeply. Keep in mind that your breaths should be low and slow. Do the "talk test." That is, can you carry on a conversation while you're engaged in your chosen activity?
- When you're tired, keep moving at whatever level you can tolerate. Plan to do more on a day when you are not so tired. Engage a friend to exercise with you to help you feel motivated.
- If you have trouble sleeping, exercise during the day to help you sleep better at night.
- Remember that exercise will provide energy gain rather than energy drain.

Pain

For many people, the most frightening part of any diagnosis is experiencing pain that is not treatable. Many people, however, undergo cancer treatment without ever having pain. If you do experience pain, you should talk to your health care team and together create a plan to manage your pain.

When pain is a result of tumors pressing on an organ, it can often be relieved by surgery to "debulk" (i.e., reduce the size or amount of) the tumor and/or by using radiation or chemotherapy to shrink the mass.

Cancer can also cause pain when it spreads into the bones and damages their structure. Frequently, treating the bone with radiation relieves this type of pain. Pain can occur when cancer presses on a nerve causing a burning, tingling, or shooting pain sensation. Certain pain medications are especially effective for nerve pain. Sometimes a nerve block, which makes the whole nerve numb, can be used to treat such a pain.

Unfortunately, cancer treatment itself can also cause pain and discomfort. Certain types of chemotherapy can cause neuropathy (numbness or tingling), which usually affects the hands or feet. Radiation or chemotherapy can cause damage to the lining of the esophagus or stomach (stomatitis), resulting in pain and discomfort.

Taking Control

The first step in being an empowered patient means knowing how to communicate about pain and how to take control of it effectively before it becomes disabling. Admitting that you are in pain is not a sign of weakness. Pain is a medical condition that can and should be treated. By talking about pain, you begin the process of controlling it.

You can describe your pain in many ways. For example, you can use adjectives like "tingling," "pressure," "cutting," or use a number scale. Rating your pain on a scale of zero (no pain) to ten (extreme pain) is a simple and effective way to explain this to your doctor. The rule of thumb is that any pain over a three needs to be treated. Each person is different in how they experience pain, so do not hesitate to talk to your doctor if you are experiencing pain (see Pain Intensity Scale).

Pain Intensity Scale										
0	1	2	3	4	5	6	7	8	9	10
No Pain				Medium Pain					Worst Pain	

Once you and your doctor have identified the reason for your pain, the next step is usually to choose the correct medication. There have been many recent improvements in pain management. There might be a period of trial and error while your health care team tries to find the right medication and dosage for you. The many medications available range in strength and may be short-acting (lasting just a few hours) or long-acting (lasting twenty-four hours or more). Pain medications might be given as pills, liquids, suppositories, skin patches, or injections.

There is a common myth about pain management that prevents many people from getting the pain control they need. The myth is that people will become addicted to pain medication. Addiction is very rare for people with cancer. In fact, less than 1 percent of people with cancer who are treated with pain medication become addicted. On the other hand, poorly managed pain will increase anxiety and distress, which will, in turn, intensify feelings of pain. That's why it is important to find a qualified professional who will provide you with a reasonable pain-management program to end pain and distress. If you're struggling with pain control, ask your doctor or nurse about how to find a pain specialist in your area.

For some people with cancer, mind-body practices such as guided imagery, relaxation and breathing exercises, biofeedback, massage, acupuncture, light exercise, music therapy, and counseling can help as well. (see Chapter 8 for more on Complementary and Alternative Therapies.)

Most patients will have complete relief of pain with appropriate management. You have a right to have your pain managed, but you need to communicate with your health care team about your symptoms. You can ask your oncologist to recommend a pain specialist if your pain is severe and previously tried treatments have not helped.

What About Side Effects from Pain Medications?

Unfortunately, pain medication can cause side effects, including nausea, drowsiness, and constipation. Most people develop tolerance to the drowsiness and nausea caused by opioids, meaning that the medication might cause these side effects at first, but they will eventually subside. Nausea might be treated with antinausea medication. If you are taking opioids for pain, you should always be on a bowel regimen; usually, a combination of a stool softener and laxative is best. If such solutions do not work, switching to a different pain medication might be necessary.

> **The Cancer Support Community's Bill of Rights for People with Cancer Pain**
>
> *I have the right to have my pain relieved by health professionals, family, friends, and others around me.*
>
> *I have the right to have my pain controlled, no matter what its cause or how severe it might or might not be.*

*I have the right to be treated with respect at all times. When I
need medication for pain, I shouldn't be treated like a drug
abuser.*

*I have the right to have the pain resulting from treatments and
procedures prevented or at least minimized.*

Infections and Fever

Infection can be one of the most serious side effects of treatment, and it
should be your goal to avoid it whenever possible. Infection can lead to
hospitalization, which can be costly and disruptive, keeping you from
your daily activities and loved ones. At its most serious, infection can
be life-threatening.

Infection can occur because many of the chemotherapy drugs that
fight cancer cells can also cause a decrease in a type of white blood
cell, called neutrophils, in the blood. Neutrophils are infection-fighting
white cells. Radiation to large bones like your spine, hips, or pelvis
could also cause a decrease in white blood cells. The condition when
your white blood count is dangerously low is called neutropenia.

Throughout your cancer treatment, your blood will be drawn and
tested frequently. While your medical team is keeping track of your
white blood cell, platelet, and red blood cell counts, it's important for
you to keep track, as well. Record your complete blood count (CBC) on
a CBC Log to assist you in monitoring this critical aspect of your care.

A fever is the body's natural response against invaders (such as viruses, bacteria, and fungi) that cause infection, and it can be an important
sign of infection. Fever that occurs when your blood counts are low is
considered a cancer care emergency, requiring prompt medical attention.
When you're receiving chemotherapy, take your temperature daily, using
a Temperature Log to track it. If you have a fever higher than 100.4°F
(38°C), call your doctor or nurse immediately, because it could be the
first, or only, sign that you have an infection.

Symptoms of Infection

The sooner you detect an infection, the more likely you'll minimize dis-
ruption to your treatment. Report these symptoms of infection to your
doctor or nurse right away:

- chills, shaking, sweating;
- cough, sore throat, shortness of breath, and/or chest pain;
- redness, warm skin, pain or swelling around a wound or catheter site (PICC line, port, or other central line);
- loose bowels or diarrhea for more than twenty-four hours;
- pain or a burning sensation during urination or pain in the back above the waist;
- unusual vaginal discharge or itching;
- mouth ulcers.

You're at high risk for neutropenia if you are receiving chemotherapy known to decrease the number of white blood cells; you already have a low white blood cell count or previously received chemotherapy or radiation; you are sixty-five or older; or you have another condition that affects your immune system.

You'll be susceptible to infection as long as you have a reduced number of white blood cells circulating in your blood stream. The period of time it takes for white blood cells to recover varies, depending on the type and dose of chemotherapy as well as on your body's own ability to replace the damaged cells.

Preventing Infection

The most important way to avoid the spread of infection-causing bacteria is to wash your hands frequently and/or to use an antibacterial, alcohol-based hand lotion. Take time to scrub your hands thoroughly, front and back, with soap and warm water (for at least fifteen seconds—the time it takes to sing "Happy Birthday"). Friction from washing and drying helps kill bacteria.

Your doctor may prescribe a white blood cell, growth-factor medication to help you produce more white blood cells and reduce the period of time you're at risk. These medications are given after every cycle of chemotherapy to stimulate the bone marrow to produce more white blood cells. White blood cell growth factors can cause achiness and some flu-like symptoms. They can also help you get your treatment as planned and at the full dose, ultimately improving your chances for a cure.

Preventing Infection

- **Stay clean.**
  Wash your hands often, especially before meals and after bowel movements. Clean your rectal area gently, but thoroughly, after each bowel movement.
- **Eat clean foods.**
  Wash fruits and vegetables carefully and avoid raw meat, raw seafood, and raw eggs.
- **Avoid infection.**
  Avoid crowds and individuals who might have diseases you can catch, such as colds, chicken pox, and the flu.
- **Avoid cuts.**
  Avoid cutting your skin: use an electric shaver instead of a razor, don't tear or cut the cuticles of your nails, and be careful when handling knives. Clean cuts and bruises with warm water, use an antiseptic ointment or cream, and cover them with a bandage.
- **Keep skin soft.**
  Use oil or lotion to soften your skin if it becomes dry and cracked.
- **Avoid pet waste.**
  Don't clean up animal waste, like the cat litter box or fish tank.

What's the Treatment for Infection?

If you develop an infection, most likely you will be treated with antibiotics. In some cases, hospitalization may be necessary. Obviously, you want to spend as little time in the hospital as possible. Working and/or managing other roles and responsibilities throughout treatment make it even more important to be vigilant about preventing infection.

Anemia

Anemia occurs when your red blood cell count is lower than normal. Hemoglobin (Hgb) is an important part of your red blood cells. At normal levels, hemoglobin supplies your body with the oxygen it needs to work properly. When hemoglobin is too low, less oxygen is delivered to your body's cells and tissues, and you may feel tired or weak.

Anemia-related fatigue is experienced by more than three-fourths of all cancer patients. Over half of these patients report that fatigue associated with anemia affects the quality of their daily lives more than any other side effect of treatment, including nausea, pain, and depression. Most important, if left untreated, severe anemia can make cancer therapy less effective, interfere with the completion of chemotherapy, strain the heart and cardiovascular system, and result in the need for red blood cell transfusions.

Anemia in cancer patients can result from many factors, including chemotherapy, radiation treatment, blood loss, and iron deficiency. Cancer treatments are designed to destroy cancer cells, but some can also kill or damage healthy cells, including red blood cells that carry oxygen throughout the body. Chemotherapy can also suppress the production of red blood cells in the bone marrow and affect kidney function, including the production of erythropoietin, which stimulates red blood cell production.

What Are the Symptoms of Anemia?

Anemia can be difficult to identify because early symptoms can be mild. If you're actively receiving treatment for cancer, you need to discuss with your oncologist or oncology nurse whether or not the treatment you're receiving affects your red blood cell count.

Report all symptoms of anemia to your doctor. Besides extreme fatigue and weakness, major symptoms of anemia can include

- shortness of breath;
- confusion or difficulty concentrating;
- dizziness or fainting;
- pale skin, including decreased pinkness of the lips, gums, lining of the eyelids, nail beds, and palms;
- rapid heartbeat;
- feeling cold;
- sadness or depression.

Sometimes, patients are hesitant to tell their doctor how tired they are because they want the doctor to see them doing well; other times, patients simply associate fatigue with "being sick," assume it's a normal part of cancer treatment, or are fearful the cancer is worsening. As a part of being an empowered patient in the management of anemia, you should be honest about the severity of your fatigue and its impact on your daily activities, and ask to have your blood counts tested. You shouldn't have to suffer unnecessarily.

How Is Anemia Treated?

Doctors diagnose anemia with the help of a medical history and blood tests, including a complete blood count (CBC) to measure the number of red blood cells and the amount of hemoglobin in the blood. Normal hemoglobin ranges are 14–18 g/dL (grams per deciliter of blood) for men and 12–16 g/dL for women.

Treatment of anemia varies depending upon the cause and extent of the condition. If your anemia is caused by chemotherapy, your doctor may prescribe injections of red blood cell growth factors to help you produce more red blood cells. Ask your doctor which option will have the least impact on your daily activities and schedule. Once you're on the recommended treatment, let your health care team know whether or not you're getting any relief.

It's important to track hemoglobin levels from your regular blood tests and compare them to your energy level. Discuss and share these observations with your medical team. Anemia-related fatigue is real. It shouldn't be ignored, as it can be treated. Talk with your doctor about what can be done to help improve your quality of life and keep your treatment on track.

Blood-Clotting Problems

Here are some action steps you can take to avoid problems related to blood clotting.

- Don't take any medicine without first checking with your doctor or nurse. This includes aspirin or aspirin-free pain relievers (including acetaminophen, ibuprofen, and any other medicines you can buy without a prescription).
- Avoid alcoholic beverages.
- Use a very soft toothbrush to clean your teeth.
- Clean your nose by blowing gently into a soft tissue.
- Take care not to cut or nick yourself when using scissors, needles, knives, or tools.
- Be careful not to burn yourself when ironing or cooking. Use padded gloves when you reach into the oven.
- Avoid contact sports and other activities that might result in injury.

> • Report any bleeding to your doctor immediately. You might need a platelet transfusion of red blood cells through an intravenous or central line in the outpatient clinic.

Gastrointestinal Side Effects

Nausea and vomiting are the side effects most associated with cancer treatment, but in the last twenty years, great strides have been made in developing medications that have significantly decreased nausea and vomiting. Ask your health care team about the plan to prevent nausea before your treatment. Be sure you understand any instructions about taking antinausea medications.

- Eat only small, light meals before your treatment; some people prefer to wait until after treatment to eat.
- Eat several small meals during the day rather than three large meals.
- Dried toast, crackers, and cereal will help to settle your stomach.
- Eat cool, bland foods (odors will trigger nausea).
- Avoid sweet, fatty, or fried foods.
- Chew food slowly and well to help with digestion.
- Drink liquids after meals to avoid feeling too full.
- Use relaxation and slow, deep breathing to help manage any wave of nausea you might experience.

Consult your doctor if nausea or vomiting becomes a problem. These symptoms can be managed, even if it takes trying several different combinations of medicines or therapeutic interventions.

Constipation and Diarrhea

Difficulty having a bowel movement is common for people undergoing cancer treatment. Keep in mind that medications, surgery, inactivity, and dietary changes are just a few of the factors that can contribute to changes in normal bowel function.

- Avoid over-the-counter stimulants to help you have a bowel movement.
- Your doctor may suggest stool softeners or stool-softener-plus-laxative combinations to prevent constipation. Another

alternative would be to take fiber supplements, but this should be cleared with your doctor first.

- Drink plenty of fluids (up to eight glasses of water a day) to help promote bowel function. If fruit juices are too sweet for you, consider preparing a drink of half-juice and half-water or squeezing a lime or lemon into your water.
- Try to avoid consuming too many caffeinated beverages. For most patients, one drink each day with caffeine such as coffee, tea, or soda is okay. Remember that caffeine is a stimulant and interferes with your ability to relax and to sleep, increases your heart rate, causes nausea and diarrhea, and decreases your appetite. It might also cause you to feel nervous and jittery.

Diarrhea is the passing of three or more watery bowel movements a day and can be a severe side effect of some cancer treatments. It is very important to manage this problem and get control of it quickly, because nutrients and body fluids are easily lost in a short period of time during treatment. If diarrhea is a side effect of your treatment, your health care team will discuss what to do, how to manage it, and when to call if it gets serious. If you have diarrhea, you should

- drink plenty of fluids;
- eat six small meals a day;
- avoid greasy, fried, fatty foods;
- avoid foods high in acid, such as tomatoes and citrus;
- consider a good, bland diet, such as the BRAT diet (bananas, rice, applesauce, and toast).

As with other side effects of treatment, you should ask for clear instructions on how to take medications to prevent or manage diarrhea, when to phone the doctor for problems, and what to expect from your treatment. Try to keep track of your bowel movements by recording them. If the number increases to six or more, that's an indication that you should contact your doctor.

Practice good hygiene by washing your hands before and after going to the bathroom, wiping your bottom with a baby wipe or a mild soap and water, patting dry carefully, and applying an emollient ointment such as zinc oxide or petroleum jelly afterward. Your doctor might also prescribe a skin barrier ointment to protect your skin. Don't take any medication to control the diarrhea without consulting your doctor first.

Managing Gastric Upset with Good Nutrition

Nutrition is an integral part of maintaining good health through treatment and beyond. There are many resources from which you can make a plan to eat well and nutritiously; for example, most cancer clinics offer dietary consults for their patients.

Six small meals are good for managing nausea and diarrhea. These meals should have adequate protein, carbohydrates, and fat to sustain your energy levels and assist in building your immune system and repairing your body. Consider alternatives to traditional meals, such as protein drinks or puddings. There are many vitamins and supplements that are available and sometimes even promoted to people with cancer. Be careful and a little wary of alternative therapies that boast impressive benefits. There are excellent resources available to help you practice caution and to be safe when considering these products—and your best resource is always to consult your health care team first.

Keeping track of the foods and situations that make gastrointestinal problems worse or better is always helpful. Generally, you should keep track of the things that work well for you and the things you need to avoid.

Mouth Sores (Mucositis)

Mouth sores can be a side effect of chemotherapy or radiation to the head and neck area. Sores can occur in your mouth, on your lips, and in your throat. In fact, sores can actually appear anywhere in the gastrointestinal lining. If mouth sores are an expected side effect with your treatment, visit your dentist before treatment begins, if possible. Inspect your mouth daily for red areas, sores, or white patches. White patches can indicate infection.

Here are a few action steps you can take if you experience mouth sores.

- Rinse your mouth after meals and before bed with a solution of baking soda (1/4 teaspoon) or salt (1/8 teaspoon) and water (1 cup).
- Brush with a soft toothbrush.
- Don't use mouthwashes that contain alcohol.

- Avoid sharp, crunchy, spicy, or citrus foods; alcoholic beverages; and tobacco products.
- Eat soft foods at room temperature.
- Try popsicles or ice chips to reduce pain.
- Contact your doctor if mouth sores are painful or are affecting your ability to eat or drink.

Hair Loss (Alopecia)

Hair loss, also known as alopecia, has long been an indicator that a person has cancer. Experiencing hair loss is a deeply personal and upsetting experience for most people. It's normal to be distressed about the loss of your hair and how it affects your appearance. Discussing your concerns with your health care team and finding ways to manage the loss is important for you to do.

Not all treatment for cancer will cause hair loss—and most hair loss isn't permanent. You should ask if your treatment causes hair loss so that you can prepare for it if it's an expected side effect. Hair loss usually begins ten to fourteen days following the first treatment; it's difficult to predict exactly how it will happen. Your hair might gradually thin or fall out in large clumps. You're also likely to lose hair all over your body at the same time. In most cases, your hair will grow back when your treatment has been completed. Many times, the texture and color of your new hair will be slightly different.

How Can I Manage Hair Loss?

If you plan to get a wig, visiting your hairdresser or wig store before you lose your hair is a good idea. That way, you can best match your hair color and texture to the wig. However, you might also choose a wig that is completely different from your natural hair.

Some insurance companies will supplement the cost of a wig, but you must submit a prescription written by your physician for a cranial or hair prosthesis. Frequently, cancer treatment centers will have "wig banks" where you can get a rehabilitated or new wig for free, or at low cost.

Alternatives to wigs include hats, scarves, and turbans. You should get into the habit of protecting your head from the sun by applying sunscreen and wearing a covering of some kind. It's also important to protect yourself from loss of body heat when the weather is cool by wearing a hat or other head covering.

Many people will choose to get a very short haircut or to shave their heads before they begin to lose their hair. In doing this, you'll have the opportunity to control how the hair loss will occur and have time to see the "new look" before anyone else.

Remember: Your hair will grow eventually back!

Can I Prevent Hair Loss?

You can't prevent hair loss, but you can take some precautions to prevent damage to your hair, such as avoiding permanents or coloring, curlers, and hair dryers on high heat settings. You should use a mild shampoo, soft hairbrushes, and mild lotions. The use of ice or other methods to prevent hair loss should be discussed with your physician. Any products suggested to you should be discussed with your doctor prior to use to avoid any possible harm.

Rashes and Other Side Effects on the Skin

Besides hair loss, treatment toxicities affecting the skin can include redness, cracking rashes, and an acne-like eruption. Hyperpigmentation, or darkening of the skin, is another side effect seen with some chemotherapies and radiation treatments. Color changes can be seen in the nails, around intravenous infusion sites, the palms of the hands and soles of the feet, and, for some, a "tanning" all over the body.

Another chemotherapy side effect, known as "hand and foot syndrome," causes a painful redness on the palms of the hands and soles of the feet. Sometimes this progresses to cracking and peeling. It's important to avoid heat or pressure in these areas to minimize the total effect. Other areas of pressure and resulting pain and redness are at the waistband and bra line. The use of water-based moisturizers is sometimes helpful in reducing the severity. Always tell your physician if you notice these skin changes.

A variety of skin rashes can be seen with cancer treatments. Many of the new biotherapies have skin side effects that can become quite severe. This acne-like rash is a result of the special way the new therapies work. Although the rash looks like acne, it is not acne and should never be treated with over-the-counter acne products. Your physician might prescribe moisturizing soap and treatments. In some cases, antibiotics are needed to prevent or treat infection as a result of the rash.

Treatments for cancer may increase your risk for skin sensitivities, and many skin problems are made worse by exposure to the sun, so continue protecting your skin from exposure to the sun by wearing sun-screen (if approved by your doctor), long-sleeved shirts and pants, and a hat. The skin side effects of some treatments can be alarming and diffi-cult to manage, so talk to your health care team as soon as one develops. If you follow your doctor's recommendations for management of any skin problems you encounter, your skin problems will clear up.

Nerve Changes (Neuropathy)

Neuropathy usually occurs when chemotherapy damages nerves. Symptoms of neuropathy can include numbness or tingling (especially in the hands and feet), loss of sensation, pain that feels like an electric shock, loss of balance, aching muscles, problems buttoning a shirt or picking up small objects, and difficulty concentrating or memory prob-lems. Neuropathy can improve after treatment is over, but sometimes persists for years. Here's what to do if you experience neuropathy.

- Always talk to your doctor or nurse about these symptoms.
- Avoid falls—walk slowly, use handrails, and wear supportive shoes.
- Avoid injuries—be cautious when using sharp objects or cooking.
- Avoid alcohol—even small amounts can make neuropathy worse.
- If you become confused, contact your health care team immediately.

Other Side Effects

You may experience many other side effects during cancer treatment, including

- loss of appetite;
- rectal soreness;
- watery or dry eyes;
- thrombosis (blood clots in a blood vessel);
- sexual concerns.

If you have concerns about how you're feeling, be sure to write them down, and bring your notes or journal with you to the doctor. You don't have to "tough it out" or pretend as if everything's all right. Cancer and its treatment bring profound challenges to you and your family. By taking charge of your treatment and any side effects you experience, you'll improve the quality of your life—and might well enhance the possibility of your recovery.

Patient Action Plan

- **Report anything unusual to your doctor.**
  Keep track of any symptoms or side effects you experience. Eventually you will know your body and learn how to manage common side effects from treatment.
- **Contact your doctor or nurse if your temperature is more than 100.4°F.**
  You might have to go to the hospital for medication and hydration.
- **Prevent nausea.**
  Ask your health care team how to prevent nausea before your treatment begins.
- **Identify needs and ask for help.**
  Family, friends, neighbors, and members of your religious community might be able to help with chores and errands, such as transportation, grocery shopping, walking the dog, weeding the garden, and housework.
- **Practice energy conservation.**
  Learn to prioritize, pace yourself, ask others for help, eliminate unnecessary tasks, modify how you do things, and avoid things that cause stress.
- **Exercise when you can and eat healthfully.**
  Consider exercise and good nutrition a priority for better long-term health and well-being.

Chapter 10

Managing Practical Matters

I had genetic testing done, but my insurance (Medicaid) said they wouldn't pay for it. It was a $5,000 test! I couldn't afford it. But I said I would be willing to make a payment plan, and they sent me the paperwork. Then I found out Medicaid picked up the test after all. It gets so confusing sometimes.

BETH,
breast cancer survivor

WHILE THE THOUGHTS of cancer patients center on health and recovery, concerns about finances, insurance, legal issues, and employment usually follow closely behind. Many cancer patients fear that the illness will drain their family's financial reserves, and they wonder whether they'll be able to continue to work or return to work. They are also unclear about what insurance coverage protections are guaranteed by law.

Seeking and paying for treatment can cause trauma that is even deeper and more disturbing to the lives of patients and caregivers than most of us imagine. The Cancer Support Community's (CSC's) Research and Training Institute released a pilot study in April 2010 that sought to quantify the distress and realities of managing cancer care. As reported in *The Wall Street Journal* (April 13, 2010), this groundbreaking report looked at the financial strains that cancer patients and their caregivers confront in seeking treatment. The financial burdens related to cancer treatment made patients and caregivers vulnerable to post-traumatic stress disorder with symptoms that included extremely high levels of anxiety, depression, and other mental health problems. We found that 81 percent of patients and 72 percent of caregivers experienced "moderate to severe" stress levels from their monetary burdens, requiring clinical intervention and/or psychological support. These stress levels were

113

even greater than that of those who witnessed the terrorist attacks in New York City on September 11th and akin to that of underprivileged, displaced survivors of Hurricane Katrina.

Many of those interviewed fell below the poverty line: 43 percent of survey respondents earned a household income of less than $40,000 a year. Individuals were mistrustful of the free programs designed to assist them, fearful that they would not qualify for them, and worried that their financial statements would be used to expose them in other ways. The trauma-related anxiety they felt interfered with, and at times made impossible, their ability to navigate the system and to access financial resources such as co-pay assistance. These overwhelming concerns also inhibited their ability to make sense of complicated information, further serving as a barrier to care. Many patients and caregivers did not obtain the support they required because of the financial costs and social stigma associated with getting help. However, what we found most surprising is that although 91 percent of the group surveyed did have health insurance, their benefits were inadequate. This speaks volumes about the need for improvements in our present health care system.

The difficulties are even greater than we had thought. While it still remains to be seen how health care reform will play out, our research is showing that the need for change is great.

Health Insurance

Health insurance coverage provides assistance with medical expenses involved in screening, diagnosing, treating, and recovering from illness. You should investigate the terms of your policy to be aware of the provisions for hospital stays, special or experimental treatments, second opinions, diagnostic measures, and long-term and/or home care. Some policies might cover nursing services or alternative health care services. Knowledge of any restrictions in the health care coverage will help avoid disappointment and unpaid medical bills. The hospital ombudsman or social worker is trained to help investigate questions with your insurance company—so seek their help.

The health care insurance industry has been in a constant state of change for the last ten years, as different types of managed care plans replace the traditional indemnity insurance that covered whichever doctor and hospital the patient visited.

Most laws governing these health insurance companies are determined by individual states and vary widely in different regions of the country. The recent addition of for-profit health care conglomerates has added to the evermore confusing picture. Currently, many rules governing Medicare, Medicaid, and "third-party payers" are under review at the state and national levels.

There's been much controversy recently about access to treatment for cancer patients. While all of us are concerned about controlling health care costs, no one wants to be denied access to appropriate testing or treatments. If payment is denied, it's best for you to work with your doctor and/or treatment facility to reapply for appropriate payments.

If these efforts fail, there are a number of reimbursement specialists that operate hotlines for various drug manufacturers—and several may even contact the insurance company directly on your behalf (see the Appendix resources for places to call for financial support).

Patient advocates, lawyers, the patient, and/or family member can also pursue claim rejections with insurers and, sometimes after a long and arduous battle, obtain payment. If all else fails, contacting your local state legislator might provide the necessary clout to gain preapproval for a needed test or treatment.

The Affordable Care Act and Why it Matters to Cancer Patients

President Obama signed the Affordable Care Act (ACA) into law in March of 2010. Although the law is not perfect, there are a number of provisions that will dramatically improve access to and quality of care cancer patients receive in this country.

With many provisions already in effect, cancer patients are finally being protected from a number of unfair insurance practices. For example, people with cancer can no longer be denied coverage due to pre-existing conditions, be charged more out of pocket simply because of their health status, face annual or lifetime caps on coverage, or be faced with impossible choices like having to spend down their life savings because coverage is unaffordable. Additionally, cancer patients in Medicare are no longer paying co-pays for proven preventive services.

In addition to these broad-based consumer protections, cancer patients will see a number of other benefits from the law over the next few years. All health plans that operate in a state's health exchange must provide coverage for a set of "essential" benefits, including appropriate cancer screenings, treatment, and follow-up care. Medicare will cover and encourage beneficiaries to get a yearly check-up to discuss disease prevention. For patients who want to take part in clinical trials, coverage will be more affordable and accessible.

The ACA is a complicated law and how the details will affect you and your family can be difficult to understand. There are ways to learn more from your health plan, your state insurance commissioner, or by visiting the Web site for the U.S. Department of Health and Human Services (HHS) at www .healthcare.gov.

Types of Health Insurance

- Health Maintenance Organizations (HMOs) provide, offer, or arrange for a wide range of health care services to cover a specified group of enrollees for a fixed, periodic prepayment. With an HMO, all costs are covered—sometimes with minimum co-pay—as long as an appropriate referral is obtained before seeking any care outside of the office of the primary provider. However, it might be difficult to obtain coverage for second or third opinions or treatment from a health care provider who is not part of that particular HMO system.
- Indemnity insurance policies are the traditional insurances in which physicians and other providers receive payment based on each billing charge for a visit or service provided. Although indemnity policies provide the best coverage in terms of flexibility, there is usually a deductible and/or co-pay required for doctor visits and medications.
- Preferred Provider Organizations (PPOs) combine some aspects of the HMO and the traditional indemnity policies. The patient may choose his or her provider from a list of "preferred providers" and does not need a referral before seeking additional opinions or treatment. However, if you make a decision to see a

provider or seek hospitalization in a center outside the network, the co-pay might be significant.

- Major medical is a plan that is usually part of the traditional indemnity insurance that pays for a percentage of expenses not covered by the hospitalization part of the plan.
- Medicare, Medicaid, and veterans' benefits: Medicare, a federal insurance program, provides coverage for testing, hospitalization, and treatments for people age sixty-five or older. Medicaid is a joint federal and state health insurance program and provides coverage for some low-income people with disabilities. People with Medicare or Medicaid coverage are usually offered managed care or indemnity (traditional) coverage plans, depending on the state in which they live. Veterans might receive benefits through the Veterans Affairs' program, in addition to coverage under other insurance programs.
- COBRA, or the Consolidated Omnibus Budget Reconciliation Act, is a federal law allowing a person to maintain insurance coverage. One might continue to be covered by his or her last employer's insurance for up to eighteen months, but he or she is responsible for paying the monthly premiums.
- Short- and long-term disability insurance might provide financial assistance when a person is being treated for cancer. An employer might carry disability insurance for employees, and/ or an individual might purchase policies from private insurance carriers.
- There are two different disability benefits available from the Social Security Administration: Social Security Disability Insurance (SSDI) and Supplemental Security Income (SSI). The medical requirements and determination process are the same under both programs. Eligibility for SSDI is based on your work history and begins six months after you are considered disabled. For people younger than sixty-five, Medicare health coverage doesn't begin for twenty-four months. SSI disability payments are made on the basis of financial need, and most people who get SSI are also eligible for food stamps and Medicaid.

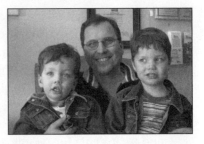

I remember thinking (upon diagnosis) that if I were to die, I would be denied the opportunity to watch my children grow up and that all the plans and dreams my wife and I had would have to go unfulfilled. Every thought I had was worse and more tragic than the last. However, even in those first few moments, one thought was able to penetrate my burgeoning sadness and provide solace and peace of mind: Though I may die, and my wife and children be emotionally devastated, at least my life insurance will assure that their lives are not destroyed.

DREW VAN DOPP,
community member, Cancer Support Community, Delmarva

Patient Assistance Programs

Patient Assistance Programs (PAPs), funded by state government, charitable organizations, and pharmaceutical companies, are available to help cover medical costs for people who are having financial difficulty. Nearly every pharmaceutical company has a PAP for many of the medications they produce. These programs provide discounted or free medication to people who qualify. Some PAPs can also facilitate an exception and/or appeal process with your insurance company for coverage of particular medications. Although there are financial criteria to qualify for PAP services, the criteria can be very generous. If you need help, it's wise to apply.

In addition to the PAPs, several nonprofit organizations have developed programs to help patients with the prescription costs including co-pays. There are several ways to get more information about co-pay assistance programs, prescription drug benefits, and how to access financial resources.

- Read *Frankly Speaking About Cancer: Coping with the Cost of Care*, a free, comprehensive resource guide available on www .cancersupportcommunity.org.
- Call the Patient Advocate Foundation (PAF) with direct

questions at 800-532-5274 or view www.patientadvocate.org.
PAF's Co-Pay Relief Program is www.copays.org.
• Ask an oncology social worker, patient navigator, or oncology
nurse at your cancer center.

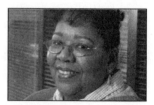

*The drug companies will give the medi-
cine for free sometimes, but only if you
apply.*

NANCY,
metastatic breast cancer survivor

Obtaining Adequate Life Insurance

The following suggestions, from *Charting The Journey: An Almanac
of Practical Resources for Cancer Survivors* by National Coalition for
Cancer Survivorship, might increase a cancer survivor's ability to obtain
adequate life insurance.

• Try large companies that carefully grade type and stage of cancer.
• Obtain estimates from several companies. An efficient way to do
this is to have an independent agent (one who does not work for
a particular company) shop among the companies in your area
to obtain the best possible plan for your needs. You can get a
list of all licensed insurance brokers in your area from the state
insurance department.
• If you are unable to obtain a life insurance policy with full death
benefits, consider a graded policy. If you die from cancer within
the first few years of the policy—usually three years—a graded
policy returns only your premium plus part of the face value
of the policy to your beneficiaries. If you die after the waiting
period has passed, the company will pay the full face of the
policy.
• Try to obtain life insurance through a group plan. Many
employers and organizations that offer group health insurance
also offer group life insurance. The insurance company does
not make an individual evaluation of the health of each plan
member of a large group; however, your health may be considered

if you participate in a plan with a small number of members (for example, if you are one of thirty workers). If your health is considered, you may be excluded from the plan, denied full benefits, or required to pay an extra premium.

The American Council on Life Insurers (www.acli.com) provides information about brokers who specialize in high-risk life insurance.

Employment and Legal Issues

While many people with cancer feel unable to continue with their normal employment during treatment, some people find it extremely valuable to maintain as much of their "normal" lifestyle as possible. If you feel able to work, there's probably no reason why you shouldn't do so.

The Americans with Disabilities Act (ADA) is a law that includes cancer as a disability with protections. The goal of the ADA is to end job discrimination against people with disabilities (including cancer), including discrimination regarding hiring, promotions, firing, pay, job training, and other aspects of work including job benefits. The Family and Medical Leave Act allows a patient or a family member caring for an ill person to take up to twelve weeks off from work without penalty or loss of benefits, but without pay.

Many cancer survivors need some physical rehabilitation before they are able to return to their old jobs or start new ones. Several different kinds of physical rehabilitation that might be helpful are

- physical therapy to gain strength and mobility;
- occupational therapy to increase strength and coordination of the body and to evaluate the ability to return to daily activities;
- rehabilitation counseling to help deal with the emotional impact of a disability.

Employment rehabilitation might be needed if you decide to seek a different kind of work than you did before cancer. You might be eligible for job retraining through the Vocational Rehabilitation Act of 1973, and there are employment agencies that can help with this process. The Office of Vocational Rehabilitation or a private employment agency can assist you in finding out about these services.

Seeking Legal Assistance

If you feel you've experienced discrimination in emp‍
ance matters, you might decide to seek the advice of a‍
case, it's highly advisable to contact a lawyer who spe‍
ment or insurance law and has experience working with people who've
had cancer.

Lawyer referral services are programs provided by a local or state bar
association to help you locate a private attorney to handle legal matters
or problems. There might be a fee for the first consultation. The referral
service might be able to help you decide whether you need to see a lawyer.

If you need a lawyer but can't afford legal fees, a useful resource is
the legal aid or legal services office in your county of residence. These
offices handle some types of legal matters for people eligible under income guidelines established for their operation.

Important Papers

Although most people with cancer recover and live for many years after their initial treatments, fears about declining health may stimulate
thoughts about wills and living wills. People have a legal and moral
right to decide which kind of medical treatment they want, or don't
want, if and when they are seriously ill and their deaths are expected.
They have a right to choose who will make decisions for them when
they are no longer able to speak or think clearly and to designate who
will get their property after they die.

A will is a legal document, usually prepared with the assistance of a
lawyer, that designates the distribution of a person's property after his or
her death. This document determines who will get the person's money
and belongings and who will be responsible for a person's underage
children in the absence of the other parent. In many states, if there's no
will, an agent of the state will make these decisions.

An advance directive is a general term that refers to your oral and
written instructions about your future medical care, in the event that
you become unable to speak for yourself. Each state regulates the use of
advance directives differently. There are two types of advance directives:
a living will and a medical power of attorney.

A living will is a type of advance directive prepared by an individual
that puts in writing his or her wishes concerning medical treatment if

me should come when he or she is no longer able to express those wishes verbally. Most states honor a living will prepared in advance by a patient; however, the laws concerning the preparation and implementation of such a document vary from state to state.

A medical power of attorney is a document that enables you to appoint someone you trust to make decisions about your medical care if you cannot make those decisions yourself. This type of advance directive might also be called a "health care proxy" or "appointment of a health care agent." The person you appoint might be called your health care agent, surrogate, attorney-in-fact, or proxy.

In many states, the person you appoint through a medical power of attorney is authorized to speak for you any time you are unable to make your own medical decisions, not just at the end of life. It's important to choose the person who's most likely to be able to carry out your wishes; sometimes a spouse or close family member isn't the best one because he or she is too emotionally involved. Be sure your proxy or agent has access to the signed directives and that your oncologist has a copy, as well. It's best to put these plans in place as soon as possible, before you become too disabled and doctors are forbidden to communicate with loved ones due to Health Insurance Portability and Accountability Act (HIPAA) privacy rules.

When it comes to handling practical matters, discussing all of your decisions with close family members, supportive friends, spiritual advisors, and health care providers will minimize confusion and help everyone involved feel more comfortable with whatever decisions you make.

You Are Not Alone

There are several organizations and Web sites that offer very practical support (please see resources in the Appendix for many more supportive organizations).

- Survivorship A to Z (www.survivorshipatoz.org) offers information on insurance, finances, government benefits, planning ahead, day-to-day living, emotional well-being, medical care, and work issues (in summary or in depth).
- Patient Advocate Foundation (PAF; www.patientadvocate .org) offers the *National Financial Resources Guidebook for Patients*, a state-by-state directory of information for patients

seeking financial relief for a broad range of needs including housing, utilities, food, transportation, medical treatment, and children's resources. PAF also offers a co-pay relief program with direct financial support to patients (www.copays.org or 866-521-3861).

- Cancer Legal Resources Center (www .disabilityrightslegalcenter.org) offers free and confidential information and resources on cancer-related legal issues for anyone coping with cancer.

The Hospice Option

Hospice enables a person to stay at home and receive pain medication, oxygen therapy, skilled nursing care, and emotional support through educating and helping the family in providing care during the last weeks of life. The term "hospice" isn't new. Hundreds of years ago, a hospice was a place of refuge for travelers, often operated by a religious order, which provided comfort, kindness, and nourishment to people in need.

Hospice is committed to assisting the patient and his or her loved ones in many different ways that traditional health care is not.

- Hospice treats the person, not the disease.
- Hospice offers palliative, rather than curative, treatment.
- Hospice addresses the physical, emotional, social, and spiritual needs of the person with cancer and his or her significant others.
- Hospice allows patients to spend their last days at home, alert and free of pain, among the people and things they love.
- Hospice emphasizes quality rather than length of life.
- Hospice offers help and support to the patient and family twenty-four hours a day, seven days a week.
- Hospice helps family members and loved ones cope with the experience of the patient's dying.

In addition, hospice provides continuing contact and support for family and friends for at least a year after the death of a loved one. Best of all, most insurance plans and Medicare cover the costs of hospice care.

Hospice care is available when your cancer has become essentially unstoppable, and your death is generally expected within six months. But many physicians and families are uncomfortable addressing this likelihood, so they put off referrals to hospice programs until a person is near death. Unfortunately, at this stage, much less can be done to help the patient and family prepare and cope—which is why it's vitally important to discuss the option of hospice as early as possible as part of your end-of-life planning.

> *It gives me comfort to prepare for when I'm no longer here, so that I've settled my affairs. I don't feel like it's a preparation for death, I feel like it's a preparation for life. My attitude is, "While I can still move, I'm going to do everything I can . . . and take advantage of the time that I do have."*
>
>

CHRIS,
metastatic breast cancer survivor

Patient Action Plan

- **Review your insurance plan to become familiar with what kind of policy it is and what it covers.**
  Call to ask questions if you have them—don't let your insurance expire.
- **Keep careful records of all expenses related to medical treatment.**
  Expenses include transportation, because major medical insurance might cover expenses not covered by the hospitalization plan. Uncovered medical expenses are tax deductible if they exceed a certain percentage of your adjusted gross income.
- **Fill out any required claim forms, and file as promptly as possible.**
  If needed, seek help in filling out forms from the doctor's office, the hospital social worker, or the home-care agency. Keep copies of paid bills.
- **If your medical and other bills begin to accumulate faster than you can pay them, don't wait for a crisis.**
  Approach your creditors to work out a payment schedule you can manage.

- **If you are changing jobs, consider your insurance needs.**
  Do not give up the insurance you have until you have determined where you will obtain future coverage.
- **Work with an experienced attorney.**
  Draft your advance directives (your living will and medical power of attorney) with a professional.
- **Tap into helpful resources.**
  These include hospice or organizations and Web sites such as Survivorship A to Z, the Patient Advocate Foundation, and the Cancer Legal Resource Center.

The Appendix of this book offers much more information about helpful resources.

Part Three

Making the Mind-Body-Spirit Connection

Chapter 11

Coping with Cancer

Having cancer transformed me very powerfully in positive ways: I don't sweat the small stuff anymore and try not to sweat the big stuff either. I have a magnet on my desk that says, "I didn't survive cancer to die of stress," and I point that out to my boss all the time.

MARILYN,
colorectal cancer survivor

N THE LAST SEVEN YEARS, as we have discussed throughout our book, the Institute of Medicine has helped bring the emotional and social needs of survivors to the forefront of cancer care. Two major reports, *From Cancer Patient to Cancer Survivor: Lost in Transition* and *Cancer Care for the Whole Patient: Meeting Psychosocial Health Needs*, focused on this important message: "Health is determined not just by biological processes but by people's emotions, behaviors, and social relationships."

Indeed, these reports provide a foundation for understanding cancer patients' emotional problems and call for changes in standards of care for treatments. Further research has reiterated that people with cancer struggle with distress as well as emotional and social problems, and that when patients address their emotional well-being along with their physical well-being, better quality of life and health outcomes are sure to follow.

What Are the Pressures?

The psychological impact of cancer varies considerably, depending on the extent of the disease and each person's situation and personality. Living with cancer and undergoing treatment can cause lifestyle disruptions, changes in family roles, a depletion of financial resources, and a decrease in self-esteem. Although emotional distress is common, it is frequently an ignored side effect of cancer. Many people hesitate to share their concerns for fear that others will see them as "weak" or having a "negative attitude." In fact, it's normal for people who are dealing with cancer to experience a whole range of emotions. Every single patient, at every stage of disease, regardless of the type of treatment, deals with issues that cause some level of distress. This can range from common feelings of vulnerability, sadness, and fear of recurrence or death to emotional reactions that are more disabling, such as clinical depression, intense anxiety, or panic. Emotional distress can affect your ability to carry out daily activities and to participate actively in your treatment. It can also worsen physical symptoms.

Side effects from cancer treatment can add to emotional distress. When they are painful or disabling and interfere with daily activities or disrupt treatment schedules, this might create even more anxiety. You might even fear that you won't be able to cope with the rigors of treatment. This is why treatment side effects and psychological well-being should be addressed simultaneously. Such a dual approach will help you maximize your ability to cope and recover. If you feel that your emotional well-being is not being addressed, you can and should ask for support.

It takes time to accept the diagnosis of cancer and to understand what it will mean for both you and your family. Everyone's reactions will differ and will probably vary over time. But you're not alone. Many other people with cancer share these feelings and concerns, and sometimes it helps to talk with other people going through treatment. By becoming an empowered patient, you can regain a sense of control about your treatment and your life, and you can find hope and meaning throughout the cancer experience.

What Are the Stages of Emotional Distress?

Before receiving your first treatment, you might feel a loss of control: you've just been diagnosed with a potentially life-threatening illness, and you don't know what's going to happen. To combat this feeling, it is important to gather as much information as possible and to find someone to talk with who has been through treatment. This will remind you that you're not alone and that you can receive the support you need.

By the middle of treatment, you might feel overwhelmed, even unable to manage daily responsibilities. This is a normal reaction, and often reflects the strain on your physical and emotional energy as you manage treatment and cope. Upon completing treatment, you might feel afraid of the unknown and abandoned by your health care team or others involved during treatment.

> • **Finding a Way to COPE***
>
> According to the *Journal of Psychosocial Oncology*, the COPE model, based on an orderly problem-solving approach, is useful for regaining a sense of control when stressed. Here's how it works. You start at the end with "E" (expert advice), and by the time you work your way back to "C" (creativity), the problem is solved.
>
> **C**–Creativity in problem-solving can be achieved with brainstorming
> **O**–Optimism, to stay focused on the positive
> **P**–Planning, to identify manageable ways to deal with your emotions or problem
> **E**–Expert information, to gather answers to your questions with the best information available
>
> *The COPE Model was originally developed by Dr. Peter Houts: *Home Care Guide for Cancer*. American College of Surgeons. 1994.

At any stage, you and your loved ones might find a support group to be beneficial in learning valuable information and feeling less alone in making the transition from being ill to living well after cancer. Abundant research validates that talking with others who understand what you are going through and receiving information in a supportive environment will help reduce distress, anxiety, and depression.

Anger is also a normal and healthy response to having cancer. It is an emotion that might arise during interactions with members of the health care system or your own family. If you, like many other people, were raised to view expressions of anger as wrong, you might feel guilty and try to deny these feelings. However, expressing anger in a productive and thoughtful manner can prevent emotions from building up and potentially leading to more serious emotional problems such as hostile, reactive, and/or impulsive behavior.

Feelings of Depression

Depression and emotional distress can make it more difficult for you to cope with the physical symptoms. Long-term distress, including depression and intense anxiety, might even affect your immune system and make it harder for your body to fight illness. Many people with cancer experience some degree of depression, but thankfully, there are also many highly effective treatments for this condition.

The first and most important step in treating depression is to recognize that a problem exists and ask for help. It becomes a problem when your emotions stop you from activities you enjoy or otherwise could or should be doing. If you think you are suffering from depression, talk to a counselor.

Measuring Distress

According to the National Comprehensive Cancer Network's (NCCN's) distress management guidelines, "Distress should be recognized, monitored, documented, and treated promptly at all stages of disease. All patients should be screened for distress at their initial visit, at appropriate intervals, and as clinically indicated especially with changes in disease status (remission, recurrence, progression). Screening should identify the level and nature of the distress. Distress should be assessed and managed according to clinical practice guidelines."

Many influential medical groups, including the American Society of Clinical Oncology, the American College of Surgeons, the NCCN, and the Institute of Medicine, have recognized that screening cancer patients for their emotional, physical, and social concerns is critical to ensuring quality care. Yet, distress screening is largely nonexistent. This is especially true in community settings (such as community hospitals and private oncology practices) where up to 85 percent of cancer patients in the United States are treated today. In fact, emotional distress is not well addressed, especially as patients transition from active treatment to their lives beyond.

In 2011, the Cancer Support Community's (CSC's) Research and Training Institute conducted a study to address this challenge and encourage the development and universal adoption of successful distress screening tools. We learned that the top five areas of distress are: fatigue, insomnia, financial difficulties, pain, and worry about the future.

Because this is a growing area of research, several distress screening tools are being developed. The CSC is validating a tool called the CancerSupportSource™, which is a tailored approach to measuring and managing an individual's level of distress. In a series of twenty-five questions, the screening tool rates concerns about issues such as sleep, bodily image, disruptions at work, worries about the future, relationships, and side effects. CancerSupportSource™ first assesses the problem, then goes one step further to identify appropriate resources for support to address the problem(s) identified. Currently, this tool is being used at several clinics and CSC affiliates across the United States. In the future, this tool will become widely available, at no cost, in community clinics, hospitals, and private practices around the country.

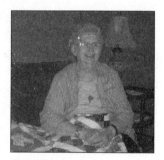

I became a member of Gilda's Club when it first opened—when I had been diagnosed with breast cancer and my husband passed away suddenly. This was the most difficult time in my life. I don't know how I would have gotten through it without Gilda's Club. The support groups, activities, and, most important the people, helped me move forward with life. As the years passed I transitioned into helping others—and being able to support others like I was supported is so rewarding!

MARY ELLEN VAN DYKE,
community member and volunteer, Gilda's Club, Metro Detroit

10 Actions You Can Take to Feel Empowered After Cancer

1. Take one step at a time.

Take a moment to slow down when you feel stressed or overwhelmed. Allow yourself to think carefully about what you need to do. You have time to gather information and make an informed decision. In fact, it's wise to ask your doctor how much time you have before you need to make a treatment decision. You might have more time than you realize.

2. **Seek support from others.**
   People often find comfort and answers when talking with others who share common experiences and challenges. Contact the organizations listed as resources throughout this book to connect with others.

3. **Communicate openly with your health care team.**
   Having an open and honest relationship with your medical team will help to increase trust and help you feel a greater sense of control. Even when your medical team includes people you've only just met, talk with them about your concerns and questions. Consider a second opinion, or even a third, and ask about clinical trials as an option (see Chapter 7).

4. **Prepare a list of questions for each appointment.**
   Ask for clarification of terms you don't understand. Ask about your options—and what each option may involve (recovery time, side effects, long- and short-term expectations). Keep notes or ask if you can record your conversation.

5. **Express your feelings.**
   Cancer and the treatment process are stressful, and they tend to trigger many strong emotions. It helps to find ways to acknowledge the range of feelings you have: journaling, support groups, or professional counseling are just a few useful strategies.

6. **Openly ask for support.**
   Friends and family often want to help, but don't know how. They will appreciate specific examples of support. Preparing meals, making phone calls for you, joining you for a movie, going with you to medical appointments to take notes, and discussing what you heard afterward are examples.

7. **Learn to relax.**
   It helps to learn how to find a calm, controlled physical state that can reduce your stress. Treat yourself. Consider a relaxation program or engage in calming activities, such as walking, yoga, reading, or music.

8. **Remember: this is *your* body.**
   Decisions about cancer treatment are very personal and they are yours to make. Do your research and develop a plan that

you feel comfortable with with your oncologist, surgeon, partner, or family member.

9. **Find a "new normal."**

A cancer diagnosis can be life changing. It can be an opportunity to reprioritize goals and reframe your self-image. Focus on living in the present and enjoying every moment with the people you care about—with appreciation for your new body.

10. **Maintain a spirit of hope.**

You might have cancer, but cancer does not have you! Remember that many people have survived a diagnosis of cancer. Draw upon your spiritual beliefs, cultural customs, and family connections. Hope can be a motivating factor in your recovery.

Stress and the Immune System

Psychoneuroimmunology (PNI) is a scientific discipline that studies the link between the mind and the body—how thoughts, feelings, and attitudes positively or negatively affect illness or health. PNI scientists propose that long-term unremitting stress reduces or diminishes the positive impact of the immune system, while positive emotions enhance the immune system. Because the first line of defense against illness or disease progression is the immune system, enhancing its power by reducing stress and increasing positive emotions—at the very least—improves your quality of life and might even enhance the possibility of recovery.

Stress-Reducing Techniques

There appear to be several ways to cope actively with cancer that not only improve quality of life, but may actually enhance immune function. These include

- managing stress through muscle relaxation, mindfulness meditation, or gentle yoga;
- utilizing problem-solving strategies like COPE (previously mentioned), especially with difficult treatment decisions;

- managing the side effects of treatment like fatigue and pain;
- managing lingering depression, and making sure that it is treated.

To reduce stress and enhance the power of your immune system, several questions come to mind.

- What are your most significant stressors?
- Which emotions are positive and should be boosted?
- Which are negative and should be diminished?
- Which stressors can be reduced?
- Who are the people in your life that you can rely on for support and care?

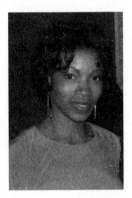

My life has not stopped because I've been diagnosed with metastatic breast cancer. I pace myself, yet I am passionate about pursuing my dreams. I consider the cancer aspect of my life as a chronic condition—a "thorn in my side"—but it will never define who I am as a woman.

KHADIJAH,
breast cancer survivor

The Expression of Emotions

Important research on emotional expression has been applied to people participating in professionally facilitated cancer support groups similar to those offered at CSC. Over the last thirty years, psychosocial oncology has aimed to incorporate new research findings into the way programs and services for emotional support are delivered.

Through psychosocial oncology research, scientists have learned that the expression of emotions is an important component for managing the diagnosis and treatment of cancer. In particular, primary negative emotions—fear, anger, and sadness—are normal and adaptive. Research has shown that the process of accessing, expressing, integrating, and reframing your emotions within a support group improves quality of life.

However, if these same emotions are repressed, they can lead to hostility, isolation, reactivity, and depression.

Planning for Death and Dying—on Your Own Terms

Death and dying is not something we want to think about, but it's certainly something that goes through everyone's mind when cancer is advanced or treatment isn't successful. It's normal to think about what will happen. Generally, a life-threatening illness prompts a re-examination of priorities, and it's helpful to prepare for whatever the future might hold. It helps to anticipate what everyone might need and want to achieve in the weeks, months, or even years ahead.

In thinking about death and dying, there are both emotional and practical issues to consider. Emotional issues related to preparing for death can include denial or anger that it is happening, depression and sadness that death is inevitable, and acceptance that death will occur. Having open, honest communication with your doctor and your family is a critical part of preparing emotionally and maintaining as much control as possible. Practical issues pertain to getting your papers in order (see Chapter 10) and to ensuring that your wishes will be carried out in the event of your death.

Although few of us like to think about it, we all know that eventually death will come. Approaching death often brings about a change in how we view life, what we value, and how we relate to the people around us. There's no right or wrong way to face the end of life—as part of your own final expression, you'll do what's right for you. However, it might be valuable for you and your loved ones to consider questions about end-of-life care together and to proceed toward the end in a way with which each of you feels comfortable.

Honest and open communication is essential. Many people with advanced disease seek the help of professional counselors, spiritual advisors, and support groups to help them cope with the feelings they have about their situations and to improve their communication with loved ones. It's important for everyone involved to have "safe places" where they can feel free to express their fears, frustrations, and concerns as the disease progresses and death becomes more imminent.

Finally, remember that even if you're okay with a potentially terminal outcome, not everyone can handle the grief and suffering of anticipated loss. Some friends might disappear, while other unexpected new sources of support might appear in your life. Stay as open as you can to all experiences—every interaction you have at this time of your life will be that much more meaningful in the end.

For Better Health, Express Yourself

Learning to express a whole range of emotions within a support group or a safe environment can lead to

- decreases in hostility;
- greater self-confidence and assertion;
- greater expressions of support, empathy, interest, and humor;
- better physical health and physiological functioning.

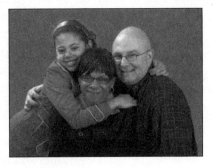

Honing these skills might enable you to balance the expression of strong emotions without alienating others—especially family and friends. I'd say, as a person who was raised to be independent, that I wasn't accustomed to leaning on anyone. With cancer, you have to let go. You have to rely on the strength and love of other people.

TERRI,
lung cancer survivor

The Challenge of the "Positive Attitude"

People with cancer have long been told that having a positive attitude increases their chances of survival. But how true is this? Is it really all that important to have a positive attitude in order to improve outcomes? And conversely, will a negative attitude mean a worse outcome or earlier death? The answer to both questions is: not necessarily.

In a 2004 study by Penelope Schofield and her colleagues at Peter MacCallum Cancer Centre in Melbourne, Australia, that involved 204 lung cancer patients, there was no evidence that a high level of optimism prior to treatment enhanced survival. However, the study underscored the importance of optimism in relation to quality of life. Those patients who were more optimistic were less depressed and more likely to adhere to treatment. Subsequent studies reiterated these findings and indicate that successful coping is not necessarily about having a positive outlook or striving for a cheery disposition. Rather, coping in a way familiar to you, which could involve anything from stress relief to exercise, can prove to be beneficial. In fact, if you're a natural curmudgeon, then continuing to be a curmudgeon might be the very thing to help lower stress; bolster the immune system; and, possibly, influence the success of your cancer treatment.

Researchers are also examining how different coping styles might affect biological indicators of disease-fighting ability such as cortisol rhythms (measures of stress levels) and natural killer cell counts (measures of immune response). With better understanding of these biological variables, there might be ways (such as muscle relaxation, stress reduction exercises, or problem-solving) to help patients manage stress and natural killer cells at levels that improve their chances of extending their lives.

People cope with stress in vastly different ways. Individuals need to identify solutions that match their natural temperaments and personalities. The next step is finding the mechanisms that enable you to keep your cortisol patterns and natural killer cells at optimum levels. In June 2010, Barbara Andersen and her colleagues at Ohio State University found not only increased survival rates but also improvements in endocrine responses and biological markers of immunity in women with breast cancer who learned muscle relaxation, problem-solving, and time-management techniques. They made dietary changes, such as reducing fat intake and increasing fiber, and exercised, all of which bolstered their ability to fight and, ultimately, survive longer.

In essence, we encourage you to develop realistic expectations about the illness so you can make good decisions about your care and not be pressured to be blindly positive. The important distinction is that optimism should not exclude sadness, anger, sorrow, grief, and hurt. You can decide to go on in the face of all of that, knowing the outcome isn't under your control.

A few good things can come from being smacked in the face with your own mortality: your priorities put in the proper order, and deep, meaningful and helpful friendships with fellow "warriors." These things can make you stronger than you ever thought possible. Don't waste precious time on energy-suckers and don't sweat the small stuff.

ALAN,
CSC online support group member

Is There a Difference Between Optimism and Hope?

Jerome Groopman, MD, author of *The Anatomy of Hope*, explains that a positive attitude or optimism refer to the thought that "everything is going to turn out for the best." But life isn't like that. Sometimes bad things happen to wonderful people. Hope, in contrast, doesn't make that assumption but rather, in a clear-eyed manner, assesses all the problems, challenges, or obstacles. Through information and education, the hopeful person seeks and finds a possible realistic path to a better future—a future that is often unknown and unknowable but is constantly reassessed based upon new information. A person with true hope will experience a wide range of emotions, including fear, anger, and sadness and will try to move forward through all the difficulties.

At the Cancer Support Community (CSC), we understand hope to be something participants gain from each other. After all, there's no person a cancer patient would rather see than a cancer survivor. The ability to make pragmatic decisions in the face of cancer based upon being with others who know what you're going through is an essential ingredient at CSC. Participants learn from each other and can increase hope, as well as reduce some of the stress associated with cancer. If longer survival is not possible, then it's reasonable to hope for other meaningful outcomes—like hoping for a peaceful death or the resolution of family conflicts. Gaining information and support from others with cancer may lead to positive immunological and stress hormone responses.

I believe that my encounter with this disease was a blessing in many ways, helping me to see what's really important in life: the love of your family, the simple pleasures of being alive, the beauty in nature, and meeting many wonderful people that I never would've known, who've become landmarks along my journey. As a result, I volunteer at CSC of Central New Jersey and at the American Cancer Society.

CHRISTINE SALEMI, *participant, Cancer Support Community, Central New Jersey*

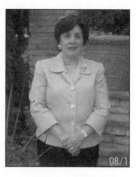

Patient Action Plan

- **Depression is a medical condition, and it can be treated.**
  It is a condition associated with a chemical imbalance in your brain. There are medications that can restore the balance and make you feel better. Depression is a very serious condition, and you should not try to deal with it on your own. It takes courage and strength to admit that you need help and to get treatment.

- **Recognize the link between stress and the immune system.**
  It's important to tell your doctor if you have feelings of depression and emotional distress. Your health care team is there to help you cope with these feelings, and to make sure that they do not have a negative impact on your immune system.

- **Express your emotions in a healthy manner.**
  Find creative ways to reduce your stress levels.

- **There are many active ways to cope with life after cancer.**
  In this chapter, we list 10 Actions You Can Take to Become Empowered After Cancer. You might be able to think of others that also suit your style.

Chapter 12

It's Not Just You

It Takes a Community

There are only four kinds of people in the world:
Those who have been caregivers;
Those who are currently caregivers;
Those who will be caregivers; and
Those who will need caregivers.

Rosalynn Carter,
Helping Yourself Help Others

aLTHOUGH RELAXATION can work wonders in helping to manage stress and side effects, nothing helps more than a strong support system. If you're blessed with close, loving caregivers and allow them to do their work to help you throughout your cancer experience, you can, and will, find the strength to keep going.

Research shows that people who are well connected to others have a lower death rate from all causes or diseases, while those who completely isolate themselves have the highest mortality rates. Therefore, connecting with caregivers as early as possible in the treatment process obviously offers a better prognosis.

But who are your caregivers? In many cases, these are the people you've known and loved your whole life. They can be spouses, close friends, neighbors, or even complete strangers. A cancer caregiver is anyone who provides physical, emotional, financial, spiritual, or logistical support to a loved one or friend with cancer. New friends that you meet who've had cancer can also become "caregivers," since meaningful interactions with people who've "been there" are often more helpful than can be expressed on paper. (For more on how to network with a support group, see Chapter 14.)

Because the journey toward wellness is not meant to be traveled alone, this chapter is for people diagnosed with cancer and their caregivers. If it takes a village to raise a child, it certainly takes a community of caring people to help a patient through the challenges of cancer.

Create a Circle of Care

You've probably said to yourself many times: "No one understands exactly what I'm going through right now." Well, then, help them understand.

Think about the people closest to you. The important thing is to let those around you help in the ways they feel they can contribute the most. Who has the personal strengths on which you feel you can rely, in good times and bad? For instance, your spouse might be best at providing emotional strength, while your sister or brother might be better suited for gathering the latest cancer news and research. Or maybe you have adult children who can help as communicators, keeping everyone in your life informed and connected when you can't or don't feel like talking. Ask for specific help, and be clear about what you need.

Allowing your family members to participate in the ways they think they can help matched with your needs will empower everyone—and such a positive experience can enhance your relationships and your well-being.

Creative Ways to Let Your Family Help

You might quickly discover that a little help can go a long way. Of course, once you're in the middle of treatments, you might be too exhausted to ask for help. That's why it makes sense to put together a list of specific ways that others can help—right now. Here's a list to get you started. Fill in every task that someone else can do to help you stay focused on taking care of yourself.

Want to Help? Here's How…	Who/When
Call or e-mail updates to others in my "circle of care." Consider using www.mylifeline.org or other sites	
Go with me to medical appointments and treatment sessions	
Do research or make calls for me (e.g., for insurance questions, medical questions, support group questions)	
Go shopping for me	
Cook my favorite foods—or things I can tolerate at this moment	
Provide child care assistance, including driving kids to school and helping them with homework	
Clean the house	
Take care of pets	
Ensure that bills are paid on time	
Do laundry	

Caregiving Basics

Becoming a caregiver can be a wonderful spiritual and emotional calling, but it can also be a challenging labor of love. Here are some basic ways to help your loved one.

- **Get the facts.**
  Learn as much as you can about the type of cancer your loved one has, including potential health issues and details regarding pain management.
- **Make connections.**
  Your local hospital likely has a medical social worker who can help you with caregiving and can connect you with a home-care course or workshop in your community. Many visiting nurse services also provide home training for caregivers. The more you know, the more secure you'll feel.

- **Encourage your loved one to manage discomfort before it gets bad.**
  Try to manage pain as it starts, so medicine won't be needed to play "catch-up." Always have sufficient medication on hand to help control pain, nausea, and other side effects of cancer treatment.

- **Keep germs away.**
  People with cancer have impaired immune systems and are more susceptible to illness. Advise sick visitors to stay home. Keep and use alcohol-based, instant hand sanitizer to minimize the spread of germs. When you need to, use latex or vinyl gloves.

- **Respect privacy.**
  Don't just barge in on your loved one—respect their need to be alone, be discreet about when to share information and with whom (always ask first), and respect their decisions. This is your loved one's body and their life.

- **Take a step back.**
  Don't assume that your loved one needs you for everything. Ask if he or she needs help before giving it. Chances are, you'll know when you're needed.

- **Fight boredom.**
  Cancer treatment and recovery often requires home rest or bed rest—but this doesn't mean you can't have fun. Help alleviate the doldrums with movies, books, tapes, and games. Sometimes even the smallest distractions can make your loved one's day better.

- **Honor quiet moments.**
  Quiet moments can be a gift. Soft music, aromatherapy (when tolerable), and warm baths offer much in the way of comfort—for both you and the patient.

- **Listen.**
  Listening and asking questions can be some of the greatest ways to take care of your loved one. Sometimes just letting them "vent" is very helpful. Other times you can speak up when your loved one is too weak, or listen to the doctor's advice when they may not be able to.

I wanted to feel like I had a job. We figured out, by trial and error, things I could do. Before a doctor's visit, I would write down the questions Marsha wanted to ask. I wouldn't ask for her—but I would take notes as we talked to the doctor. All of that turned out to be helpful. And it would amaze me, we would walk out and Marsha would have no memory of what the doctor said just ten seconds ago.

MARK,
husband of breast cancer survivor Marsha

Caregivers Can Help with Medical Discussions

Caregivers play a vital role in dealing with medical professionals—both on their behalf and in support of you. If you ask a loved one to serve as the liaison between you and your medical team, it becomes quite important to develop a positive working relationship with the health care professionals involved.

We suggest you build a "positive partnership" between your medical team and your loved one. Your caregiver can review Chapter 2 and take the following steps.

- **Ask questions.**
  Carry a notebook to every doctor's appointment and hospital stay. Jot down questions as they occur to you or your loved one. Keep a record of treatment experiences—both positive and negative. Be ready to talk to the doctor when the patient provides permission.
- **Take notes.**
  When the patient is seen by the doctor, keep notes on what was said to help manage expectations relating to treatment, side effects, and general wellness. Keep details on who or when to call in the event of an emergency.
- **Relieve discomfort.**
  One of the most difficult moments in the caregiving process is when the patient/your loved one is in pain. Naturally, you want to do something—anything—as quickly as possible to help. But nurses and doctors have many patients in their care and aren't always able to respond immediately to your needs. Try not to be upset with them once they do respond. Voice concerns outside of the

patient's presence. Ask nurses what you can do to help your loved one to be more comfortable.

• **Share hunches.**
Often, as the person closest to the patient, you become aware of issues or changes before the medical team realizes they exist. If something doesn't seem right to you, there's a good chance it isn't. Be ready to share any hunches regarding your loved one's well-being. Remember, you are the patient's advocate—and in some cases, you may be your loved one's only voice.

Most medical professionals respect caregivers who can advocate for the best care possible for their loved one. But they don't always have time for long discussions. Take a deep breath, pull out your notes or question list, and stay focused when discussing your loved one's care. Remember: you're all working together on the same team.

> *Life is no less beautiful, and everything you have to offer is no less diminished because you have cancer. I would recommend that you find opportunities to grow closer, and absolutely do NOT be afraid. Fear kills your spirit, it doesn't help your children; it doesn't help your family lift itself up. Be brave, get support, don't be afraid to lean on everyone else and know that you'll come through it.*
>
> TERRI,
> *breast cancer survivor*

A Note for Caregivers

If you are caring for someone, remember that taking time for yourself is not selfish. You need time to recharge your energies and to avoid depression and/or burnout. Your loved one will benefit from being with you when you have a healthy balance of your own. Cancer Support Community online research from 2007 illustrates that 80 percent of caregivers surveyed said that they endured regular stress and anxiety. They neglected getting regular care for their own chronic illness and suffered worse health outcomes for their medical conditions. Just like on an airplane when you are told to put your oxygen mask on before putting it on a child, caregivers must remember to take care of themselves first—so they can become better caregivers.

Talk Is Good

In general, it is important to keep the lines of communication with your family as open as possible for the duration of your cancer treatment. Doing so will not only help you keep your emotions in check, but it will also help your family to understand where you are in the process of dealing with your disease and where you could use help.

Bottling up your feelings because you don't want to bring anyone else down is understandable at first, especially when you need time to process everything that's happening to your body. But once you regain your footing, it's important to communicate as openly as possible with your caregiver as well as your entire family. After all, their minds have been working overtime, too. Sharing your worries, fears, and concerns, as well as your hopes for the future, can be a positive bonding experience for all involved.

In an effort to pin down the sometimes swirling thoughts or ideas you experience, it might help to keep a notebook of things you'd like to discuss with your family. Sometimes, just having a list can bring you both the comfort and confidence necessary to open up—especially if you tend to be a shy or private person.

The first time you have a discussion with family might be the most challenging. If you don't know where to start, use your list, or ask someone else to start talking about his or her feelings first. It won't be long before you're having one of the most real conversations you've ever shared as a group. Once you're done, celebrate this achievement for your family—moments like these will become anchors for all of you as you travel this new road together.

We were fortunate to have a great oncology nurse who was constantly giving us information. More so than the doctor. I wish our doctor (who told my wife she had melanoma) would have referred her to a support group, because it's not the end of the world. There is treatment—but you 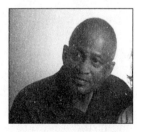 *need someone to talk to who's been there and support groups are great for that.*

OTIS,
caregiver

Helping Children Understand

One of the toughest challenges for cancer patients with children in their lives is how and when to tell them about the cancer—even if the children in question are now adults. Let's face it, nothing in your role as a parent, grandparent, aunt, uncle, or family friend has prepared you for a challenge like this one.

However much you wish you could keep it "away from the children," cancer is an impossible secret to keep. Kids overhear phone conversations, feel their parents' anxiety, and imagine the worst possible scenarios when left to their own interpretations of what's going on. Adult children notice a growing distance in your relationship.

When a parent has cancer, the natural desire to protect the children usually backfires and makes things worse. If parents don't explain the situation with age-appropriate facts, their children might

- hear about a parent's cancer from someone else and have trouble trusting their parents afterward;
- think their parents are trying to conceal something and have trouble believing the truth when they are told;
- decide that whatever is happening is too terrible to be discussed, which can isolate them from the family;
- believe that they are to blame for the cancer because they have been angry with their mom or dad;
- worry that cancer is contagious, that everyone dies from it, or that they or the other parent will get it.

Younger children need to be told that it isn't their fault and that cancer is not caused by their own negative behavior. Older children need to be given the chance to be part of the treatment and healing process, or they might feel resentful later on when you really need their support.

Children mirror the emotions of the adults around them. Therefore, how a child reacts depends very much on how well the parents or other close adults are dealing with their own feelings. School-aged children might find it hard to accept new expectations for help with younger siblings and household chores. Children of all ages fear the cancer will lead to the loss of the parent. Difficulty in discussing these issues may create distance in relationships that were once close—and this could lead to life-long behavioral issues and emotional disorders.

Sometimes, unable to fully express their fears or feelings, kids act out their emotional distress. For example, older kids might engage in risky behavior, using drugs, alcohol, or sex as a coping mechanism. If you notice that things aren't right with your child, call the pediatrician, school guidance counselor, or medical social work/counseling staff at your treatment hospital. Let any or all of these professionals recommend a counselor who's experienced in working with children whose parents have a chronic illness. Many community organizations, including the Cancer Support Community (CSC), also offer special programs like Kid Support or CLIMB for kids who have a parent with cancer. With children, in particular, open communication is the best strategy.

Don't Let Family and Friends Abandon You

As unbelievable as it might seem, sometimes family and friends abandon people with cancer. That abandonment can be physical (i.e., staying away) or emotional (i.e., distant, distracted, or unavailable). None of these responses to cancer are unusual, but let's look at how you can avoid unwanted loneliness, because it's an unpleasant situation that can literally depress your immune system.

If you've experienced a significant change in your relationships since your diagnosis—if your friends and family seem more distant than before—it's probably not because they don't love you anymore. It's much more likely that they are simply uncomfortable around people with cancer, feeling inadequate or unable to say or do "the right thing."

I got through this terrible time with the help of my wife and my daughters, who were just wonderful. My wife and I are so thankful for our daughters' help....My wife had her right cancerous kidney removed five days before my surgery. Without 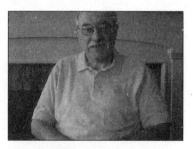 *their help, I don't know how we would have managed.*

GILBERT OSSANDON,
participant, Cancer Support Community, Central New Jersey

Reasons Family and Friends May Seem Distant

- They can't bear to be with someone they care for when that person is suffering.
- They can't bear to be with someone they care for who they fear might die.
- Being with the person who has cancer reminds them of their own vulnerability and mortality.
- They have an irrational fear that cancer is somehow contagious.
- They want to help but feel inadequate or helpless themselves.

We suggest two ways to reach out for social support. First, talk to your friends and family directly and openly about the subject of your cancer. Ask for their help, and remind them that although you have cancer now, you are still you, and you want to help the relationship to go on as it's always been. Second, ask your family and friends how you've changed since your diagnosis. Maybe there's something different about you that's causing them to stay away.

Chances are your loved ones want to be helpful; they don't want to abandon you. They just don't know how to talk or act with you now—and they finally might find this reaction frightening. This reaction can be disruptive for everyone. It's a time of confusion and emotional distress. Talking just as openly as you used to will go a long way toward helping everyone work through their fears, restoring the positive and sustaining feelings in your relationships. You might also be grateful at this time for the new friends and support you gain.

When to Seek Professional Help

Your cancer experience offers the learning opportunity of a lifetime—for all the members of your family, including yourself. Be the example; lead the way for your children as you embark on this experience together.

If, despite your best efforts, things still don't seem to be working for you or those close to you, it might be time to call a mental health expert. Counseling can help people with cancer and their family members

- learn more effective ways to communicate about the illness;
- cope better with the normal feelings and reactions to cancer;

- address changes in roles and family routines that may result;
- relieve some of the emotional and physical side effects of the cancer and your treatments. (See the Appendix for resources and information on the Cancer Support Community and its affiliate locations.)

You might ask your health care team for a referral, or share your feelings with a member of your clergy. You can determine which type of counselor will work best for your situation—the only bad choice is no choice.

Joining Hands

The cancer journey is not one you should attempt alone. Involving others in decision-making and treatment, as well as general care, can ease the stress of dealing with your cancer—offering you added health benefits that could even extend your life.

Cancer is not a solitary disease; it's an illness that affects everyone who cares about you as well. So, reach out and join hands to form a "circle of care." You'll be amazed—and blessed—by the results.

> ### Patient Action Plan for Caregivers
> Here are some considerations for a caregiver who wants to help.
>
> - **Don't try to be everything to everybody.**
>   You can't do it all—at least not right now. Forget about keeping your house, car, kids, job, pets, friendships, etc., in the manner to which they—and you—have been accustomed. You might be in crisis mode at times—and others need to understand and work with you to keep things moving.
> - **Prioritize.**
>   There are three main priorities: (1) your loved one and his or her needs with respect to the cancer, (2) you and your immediate family, and (3) your finances. Everything else will have to wait until you have time to deal with it.
> - **Delegate.**
>   Delegate every responsibility you can. Remember that most people say, "Is there anything I can do?" because they want

to help but don't know what's needed. Show them your list or your loved ones' list; keep it near you at all times so that you can pencil in tasks to assign.

- **Get or stay connected.**
  Join and participate in support groups for caregivers. If you can't get out to a group meeting, buddy up with another caregiver to share tips and experiences, or join an online support group, such as those provided by the Cancer Support Community. If you have a lot of family members who want daily reports on the patient's progress, consider starting an online group or blog to make daily postings on Web sites like www.mylifeline.org. That way, you'll only need to capture experiences once, and others can chat amongst themselves as you conserve your energy to care for your loved one.

- **Spend ten to thirty minutes a day on yourself.**
  Make sure you get a regular break by scheduling time for others to care for your loved one. Ten minutes just looking out of a window at snow, birds, trees, or the ocean will help to keep you sane. Listen to music, or go for a walk. Watch a favorite show or read a book in a place that's away from your loved one. The important thing is to reconnect with anything that makes you feel human again. You'll feel better and bring more positive energy back into the room—and you'll also have more to discuss than just the cancer. That's something your loved one will surely appreciate.

Chapter 13

Spirituality and Looking Inward

Our lives change all the time. The difference between the good changes and the bad changes is choice. But once you know this part of your life, you have to stay strong and say, "Okay, this is what I'm going to do." Maybe you can't do something that you used to be able to do. Maybe there is some- 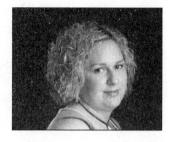 *thing that you've never tried, and you've got to go for it. You may fail, but it brings everything into focus: what's important, and what's not important.*

JORDAN,
breast cancer survivor

ATIONAL SURVEYS consistently find that religion and spirituality are important to most individuals in the Unites States. More than 90 percent of adults express a belief in God, and a little more than 70 percent surveyed identified religion as one of the most important influences in their lives. Research consistently shows that patients and family members often rely on spirituality and religion to help them deal with serious physical illnesses. They want their spiritual and religious needs and concerns understood and addressed by medical staff.

Whether or not we participate in a religious tradition, each of us holds beliefs about life, its meaning, and its value. Feeling a sense of purpose and connection to a larger reality beyond oneself can provide comfort while facing the challenges of cancer and can help you to put your situation into perspective. A spiritual life through prayer, meditation, and other practices can ease distress and be restorative, whether experienced in a religious institution or outdoors in nature or through dance, music, or other forms of self-expression.

If you or a loved one is diagnosed with cancer, you might find comfort in your spiritual beliefs—or you might question your faith. Many people ask, "Why is this happening to me?" or "Why am I being punished?" In spite of current research about the multiple causes of cancer, the belief that the illness is a punishment for some past sin or lack of faith continues to plague some patients and their families. Know that you are not to blame for your cancer. An effective way to address such painful thoughts is to work with a religious or spiritual teacher who understands you. This person might help you find a more effective way of dealing with your loss of faith. Over time, you might find a way to be more compassionate with yourself in face of all the complexity of being diagnosed and treated for your illness.

Evaluating Your Life

Being diagnosed with a potentially life-threatening disease often forces people to take a reflective look at their lives. Some might conclude that they have not accomplished enough, loved enough, or contributed enough to the world. Others might feel satisfied with where they are and what they have accomplished. The crisis of cancer can serve to help people gain insights into their beliefs and experiences and, thereby, promote personal growth.

People with cancer who have a religious affiliation can find it useful to meet with a representative of their faith, such as a minister, priest, rabbi, or other clerical person or respected member of the religious community. This "religious guide" might help you search for answers to difficult questions of faith that often arise. It can be reassuring to remember that having doubts or being angry is a normal response to facing cancer and its resulting changes.

You might be able to meet with a pastoral counselor in the hospital or through a community-based counseling agency. Because not everyone is experienced in the emotional and spiritual issues you might face when dealing with cancer, seek out someone else if the person you contact doesn't meet your needs. Hospice programs also provide spiritual counseling. These services are usually available to the community free of charge.

Members of religious and spiritual communities might also provide practical help, such as assistance with transportation, meals, visitation services, and emotional support.

The Power of Faith and Prayer

If prayer has helped you deal with other troubles, it will probably be comforting now and might help you feel less alone. Prayer and scientifically tested cancer treatments can coexist, and there's some evidence to suggest that spiritual practices, such as prayer, can assist in medical treatment, for example, by reducing hospital stays and increasing quality of life.

Medical professionals are also beginning to make a stronger connection between spirituality and medical treatment. Andrew Weil, MD, author and founder of the Center for Integrative Medicine, writes: "It's obvious to me that grief and depression impair resistance and health in general, so I would not be surprised to learn that mental and spiritual imbalances make people more susceptible to cancer. Working to improve mental/spiritual health...cannot fail to bolster defenses against all kinds of disease, including cancer."

Because having a sense of life's meaning beyond oneself can help improve your quality of life and provide inner peace, strengthen your spirit in whatever ways work best for you. Some activities that can be helpful include: prayer, meditation, reading spiritual writings, attending religious services, helping others, doing yoga, surrounding yourself with nature, listening to music, and spending time with loved ones.

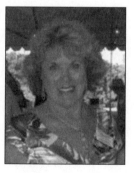

I feel truly blessed. Cancer was my wake-up call. I cannot imagine the wonderful friends and love I have received over the past years would have been a part of my life without having had cancer.

JUDITH OPDAHL,
former community member and current Executive Director, Cancer Support Community, Redondo Beach

Affirmation: Saying Is Believing

A powerful tool for framing a positive outcome, affirmation is the art of creating positive thoughts that help you to see beyond your situation and act "as if." These thoughts are useful in helping you to maintain a strong sense of control over your illness, but they can also serve as the seeds of self-fulfilling prophecy.

Because there's great benefit in repetition, affirmations work best when used daily and when strategically placed throughout your home or office so that you are reminded of them often. You might use some affirmations from a book or create your own using this list from the Cancer Support Community as a starting point.

> *I continue to be a healthy person with a joyous life.*
> *I lovingly care for myself every step of the way.*
> *I embrace every opportunity for healing that I encounter along my path.*
> *My spirit looks exactly the same, regardless of the changes in my body.*
> *I am safe and whole and open to new possibilities in my life.*
> *I continue to participate fully in as many activities as I choose.*
> *Everything is happening for my highest good.*
> *I am the creator of my own health and happiness.*
> *I am in complete control of all of my options and will make all the right decisions regarding my treatment and care.*
> *I am truly grateful for all that I have and all that I am.*

Connecting with Your Personal Source of Happiness

Whether or not you are faith-oriented and pray regularly, there's always another way to express your deepest hopes, fears, and feelings—safely and creatively. You can draw, paint, or write in a journal. Or perhaps you can express yourself with music or quiet walks in the park.

However you choose to connect with your powerful inner soul, if you do so with hope and optimism about the future, whatever it may hold, you will be a much happier—and healthier—human being. And that's exactly what it will take to help fight your cancer and increase your potential for long-term survival.

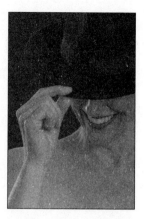

My whole life has prepared me to walk this journey and my connections with everyone at Cancer Support Community have been a treasured part of my preparation. Participating in their numerous Community Events offered me the opportunity to speak with individuals going through treatment. Playing harp through their Music for Recovery Program opened the doors for me to play in chemotherapy infusion units and patient waiting areas. Developing friendships with Charli, Kevin, and others gave me the confidence to walk this journey in my own way... through love.

AMY CAMIE,
*community member, Cancer Support Community,
Greater St. Louis*

Patient Action Plan

- **To help you deal with negative emotions, look inward—or reach outward.**
  Connect with what resonates or inspires you on a spiritual level.
- **Evaluate the quality of your life.**
  Focus your energy on the good that you have shared with others, as this kind of sharing is what connects you with the healing love of others.
- **Practice the power of prayer.**
  Even if it's just allowing others to pray for you.
- **Learn to use affirmations in your daily life.**
  One way to do that is to write and post healing quotations or thoughts around the house or office—in places where you will see them every day.

Part Four

Moving from Patient to Survivor

Chapter 14

Help Yourself, Help Others
Emotional Support, Information, and Action

*If I had not gone through those red doors of Gilda's Club, I would
have been very isolated and it would have been a very hard struggle.*

COMMUNITY MEMBER,
Gilda's Club, Desert Cities

MAGINE YOURSELF sitting in a room with ten other people who
have cancer. Just last week, your doctor suggested you attend such
a gathering. So, here you are—a new member of a cancer support
group. It begins with the professional facilitator asking you if you
would like to share anything about your cancer experience. Perhaps
you talk about what type of cancer you have, when you were diagnosed, and what treatments you're going through. You might choose
to add something about your feelings since cancer impacted your life.
In the moment before you answer, you might pause and reflect: "Why
am I here? Will participating in a support group really help me—and
if so, how?"

The Powerful Impact of Social Support

A support group is a *group* of people who meet regularly to *support*
or sustain each other by discussing problems affecting them in common. For the last thirty years, there has been extensive research on the
positive impact of support groups on the lives of people who participate as a means to cope with cancer. Research from the Cancer Support
Community (CSC) has shown that support groups help reduce the three
most significant stressors associated with cancer: unwanted aloneness,
loss of control, and loss of hope.

163

In controlled studies in a formal clinical setting, research from Stanford University and the University of California, Los Angeles, found that distress and pain were significantly reduced for women in breast cancer support groups, which led to quality of life improvements such as diminished depression and anxiety. In another study, Pamela J. Goodwin, MD, and her colleagues found that although women in professionally facilitated support groups did not survive longer, they, too, were less distressed and suffered less pain. Encouragingly, in 2010, Barbara Andersen, PhD, and her colleagues at Ohio State University found that if psychological interventions are offered early, they might provide enduring benefits and possibly extend survival. Her intervention included relaxation training, positive ways to cope with stress and cancer-related difficulties (e.g., fatigue), methods to maximize social support, strategies for improving health behaviors (diet, exercise), and adherence to cancer treatments. Eleven years after using Andersen's methods, the women who had received the treatment experienced a reduced risk of breast cancer recurrence and breast cancer death.

Community-based cancer support programs also lend further evidence that support groups can be beneficial. Results show that participants generally rate their experience as positive and helpful. A study comparing the university/clinical setting with community support groups at CSC affiliates shows that in both settings, participants had less depression and fewer trauma symptoms. They reported having better social support, feeling better able to cope with their illness, and finding greater meaning in their lives.

All in all, this is encouraging news for people participating in professionally facilitated cancer support groups—especially at CSC, with its wide geographic reach.

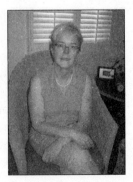

It was nearly a year ago that I first came to The Wellness Community (now the Cancer Support Community). Newly diagnosed with cancer of unknown primary, I stood at the door, looking for hope. A light rain was falling, and I was having difficulty finding the strength to open the door and enter. I stood on the steps crying, thinking how unfair this all was, and that once I entered, I

would truly admit that I had cancer. As I tried to compose myself, I heard a voice from inside. The voice said, "I don't know why you're crying, but I can't help you until you step inside." The door opened, and I became a participant (that day).

BETH BOOKER,
community member, Cancer Support Community, East Tennessee

The Cancer Support Community's Model

Based on our research, the CSC's program involves a strong social component through support groups; educational workshops; and exercise, relaxation, and nutrition programs. All of CSC's services have been developed as part of the patient empowerment model where people are:

- making active choices in their recovery;
- making changes in their lives that they think are important;
- partnering with their physicians;
- accessing resources;
- developing new attitudes toward the illness.

The CSC support and empowerment model is making a major impact on improving the lives of millions of people affected by cancer.

The Internet and Cancer Support

The Internet has certainly changed people's relationship with information and with each other. Although doctors, nurses, and other health professionals continue to be the first choice for most of us with health concerns, the Pew Internet & American Life project found that online resources, including advice from peers, have become a significant source of health information.

As broadband, wireless, and mobile access spreads, more people have the ability—and increasingly, the habit—of sharing what they are doing, thinking, or feeling instantaneously. In health care, this translates to posting reviews of medical treatments, doctors, and even health conditions. These are becoming mainstream activities, where groups of highly motivated patients and caregivers are taking an active role in tracking and sharing what they've learned.

In addition, more and more people with cancer who are too ill or live too far from support services in the hospital, clinic, or community setting can receive help at home via the Internet by participating in online support groups. An increasing body of research now supports its value.

A Growing Trend

To capture the immensity of this health-information revolution, consider the following facts.

- The Social Life of Health Information (pewinternet.org, May 2011) shows that more than 80 percent of Internet users have looked online for information about any of 15 health topics, such as a specific disease or treatment. This translates to 59 percent of all adults.
- Striking information about the extent of peer-to-peer help among people living with chronic conditions shows that: One in four Internet users living with cancer or another chronic ailment has gone online to find others with similar health concerns. By contrast, 15 percent of Internet users who report no chronic conditions have sought such help online.
- More than 24 percent of Internet users (18 percent of adults), have consulted online reviews of particular drugs or medical treatments.
- More than 16 percent of Internet users (12 percent of adults) have consulted online rankings or reviews of doctors or other providers, and 15 percent have consulted online rankings or reviews of hospitals or other medical facilities.

Do Online Support Groups Really Help?

In 2003, a study found that women who participated in professionally facilitated online support groups scheduled in "real time" experienced significant decreases in depression and negative reactions to pain, as well as significant increases in zest for life and spirituality. Another study of professionally moderated support groups that were not in "real time," but included semi-structured topics, also showed that participants experienced decreases in depression, perceived stress, and cancer-related trauma. It appears that those who join many types of online support groups are receiving mental health benefits.

The CSC offers The Living Room (originally called "The Virtual Wellness Community") at www.cancersupportcommunity.org. The Living Room is an online community where you can connect with others 24/7 about your cancer experience. The site mirrors a physical CSC location and provides free, professionally moderated support groups. It hosts physician lectures by Webcast, mind-body programs, and other services. The Living Room has received nearly 10 million hits since its introduction and nearly 1 million unique visitors. The brick-and-mortar CSCs create home-like settings for their participants; The Living Room does the same online. There's a relaxation and visualization space, a library of resources, and a kitchen filled with nutrition information.

The Living Room is open to all people, no matter what their diagnosis. This site is also useful to caregivers and children of a parent with cancer. Key features include:

- *Online Support Groups.* These groups meet online in a text-based chat room for 90 minutes each week and are facilitated by professionals specially trained to manage the diverse interactions of an online support group. We offer groups for people with cancer, caregivers, and those dealing with bereavement. In addition to the weekly meetings, each online group has its own bulletin board available 24/7 exclusively for members of that group.
- *Discussion Groups.* Discussion groups are available 24/7 and cover a variety of topics. When participating in a discussion group, you can give advice and support as well as receive help from others.
- *mylifeline.org.* You can create a personal Web site at mylifeline .org to easily build your online support community and share information with friends and family. Your personal Web site will allow you to communicate easily and receive the vital help you need during and beyond your cancer treatment. You can blog and post videos and pictures to tell your friends and family how they can support you and more.

- *Podcasts/Internet Radio. Frankly Speaking About Cancer*, the first Internet Talk Radio show on Voice America™ Network's Health & Wellness Channel, focuses specifically on how to live a better life with cancer. The show features physicians, researchers, celebrities, patients, survivors, and caregivers and offers news on cancer developments and tools that anyone affected by the disease can use to live well. The shows are available at www.voiceamerica.com or www.cancersupportcommunity.org/MainMenu/About-Cancer/Frankly-Speaking-About-Cancer/Internet-Radio-Show.

One caveat: Although there are a multitude of places on the Internet to find information and engage in discussion with other survivors, it's important to be careful about what information you may be receiving. Ask if online support group or chat room sessions are professionally facilitated or monitored; that can ensure you've found a safe environment to share information and feelings.

Key Features . . . with Lots of Benefits

The main features of The Living Room's online support groups (www.cancersupportcommunity.org) are that they

- meet weekly at a scheduled time for 90 minutes with no more than eight participants;
- are facilitated by licensed professionals trained in the Cancer Support Community's patient empowerment model;
- offer downloadable relaxation/meditation sessions, as well as sessions with speakers of note;
- are available to anyone impacted by cancer, anywhere—from the comfort of a location of your choice—without any travel requirements;
- have similar program services in Spanish (espanol .cancersupportcommunity.org).

Online and Face-to-Face Support Groups Offer Similar Benefits

You might be wondering whether it's better for you to join a face-to-face support group or one that exists online. Our research has shown that both of these settings can be helpful to you depending on your needs, geographic location, and family support network. Both types of groups offer several benefits.

- **They restore feelings of hope.**
  In a support group you'll communicate with others who are coping with cancer. In your support group, you'll find that there's always hope. Hope can give you a sense that life's worth living, and there's a reason to go on, even if you're in the final stages of the disease.

- **They reduce feelings of unwanted aloneness.**
  Support groups create opportunities to address the unwanted aloneness brought about by a cancer diagnosis by providing a safe, caring community of support. Learning that you're not alone by connecting with others who have had, or are facing, cancer can help you gain insight and understanding into your own perceptions and concerns. No matter how loved and supported by family and friends you feel, it's normal to feel as if no one really understands unless he or she has been through it personally—hence, the value of being in an online or in-person support group.

- **They help you gain a sense of control.**
  Participating in any support group can empower you to regain and maintain as much control of your life as you can. When people in your group share information, life experiences, and concerns, together you can explore ways to regain control. This helps you improve both your quality of life and your ability to solve problems.

Support Group Guidelines

Many participants make lasting friendships, reduce their stress and anxiety, and improve their awareness of services and resources while participating in our support groups. Some important guidelines have helped make CSC support groups a productive experience for those involved.

- It's important to make a commitment to attend group every week you're able. Countless participants have shared that regular attendance improves the overall group experience.

- You should arrive on time for the group. Showing up late or missing group frequently might be an indication that group support isn't the right approach for you.
- Try to stay for the entire session, or if you're participating online, participate in a way that will not lead to distractions.
- It's important to be as open as possible. The more you share, the better you'll feel and the more support you'll gain from others in the group. If you find it difficult to open up, that's fine too. Take your time to feel comfortable enough to share.

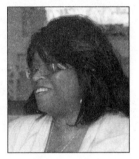

You know what's been most important to me? It was meeting people who were long-term survivors at Gilda's Club. I am so honored to know these women. It just speaks to my heart and gives me pleasure because I know there is a future.

SANDY,
breast cancer survivor

Sharing and Caring

People who are willing to share their experiences, thoughts, and feelings tend to receive more benefit from being in a group than those who don't. This type of sharing of oneself is an important way to build feelings of closeness and camaraderie. Support groups should be the one place where you don't have to pretend, hold back, or feel you must protect others from your fears and anxieties.

Being "New" to a Support Group

When you're new to a support group, you might feel anxious about what to do or how to act. After a very short time, though, you'll probably feel like "one of the family." In general, people are often surprised at how comfortable they quickly become, even if they never saw themselves before as a "support group" kind of person.

We suggest that you try participating in a group for at least three or four weeks before deciding whether or not it's right for you. If, after attending several sessions, you feel that the group doesn't meet your needs, don't hesitate to speak up. It's always best to be open with your group members about your concerns, as they might be able to help you figure out what's best for you.

We recognize that support groups aren't for everyone. Remember, there are a variety of ways to be an empowered patient, both at CSC and elsewhere.

Feeling Safe

CSC facilitators are trained to help the group establish the meeting's framework and provide a safe, compassionate environment for people to connect with one another in productive and meaningful ways. Facilitators will share in the discussions, as appropriate, and include some of their personal views, feelings, and concerns. They are experienced at understanding how groups work effectively, as well as in the aims and goals of each individual, but also know that you are far more knowledgeable about navigating your cancer and the effect it has had on your life.

As a cancer patient, you're the real expert. You know more about your life and what to do with it than anyone else in the world. Every decision you make about your life will be the right one for you. The facilitator and your group members are there to help you look at the issues, ask the hard questions, and make the difficult decisions—not to make them for you. It's the expertise of your personal experience that you bring to share with the group as a whole. In doing so, you not only help yourself, but you also discover how much you can help others.

Patient Action Plan

- **Consider the benefits of support groups in general, and seek out a group that might help you personally.**
  Ask the oncology nurse or oncology social worker at your hospital or your doctor to connect you with a group; or see if there's a Cancer Support Community resource for you. The American Cancer Society also has a great search tool for support groups at www.cancer.org.

- **Become more interested in the lives of your group members.**
  The more interested you are in them, the more interested they'll be in you. This unique friendship is built on shared experiences and can serve as an antidote to unwanted aloneness. Even if you don't feel like it, consider taking a chance to share your thoughts and concerns to see if it's helpful.
- **Take an active part in group discussions by asking questions and giving feedback.**
  This enhances how you can relate more meaningfully with others, thereby strengthening the value—both personal and for the group—of the time you spend together.
- **Get to know the members of your group as individuals through phone calls, e-mails, or in any other mutually agreeable way.**
  Let other members of the group know whether you want to be contacted. Discuss your limits.
- **Participate actively in your group, but at your own pace.**
  Warming up to new people is easier for some people than for others. If simply getting online and listening to others works for you, then start with that, and get comfortable with being in a group experience.

Chapter 15

Wellness Inside and Out:
Nutrition and Exercise*

*Adapted from material written by Carolyn Katzin, MS, CNS, MNT and Cancer Transitions: Moving Beyond Treatment™, a program developed by CSC, in partnership with LIVESTRONG

I cannot change the fact that I got cancer, but I can control how I allow cancer to change my life.

PAM,
cancer survivor

GOOD DIET and an exercise plan are especially important during cancer because your body needs additional nutrients and energy and strength to fight the disease and to heal from the disease and treatments. However, it is often challenging to eat well when you are dealing with a diagnosis of cancer, and it's even more difficult to exercise when you're tired or hurting.

After treatment, many people don't feel like eating for a variety of reasons, such as the side effects of the treatments; emotional factors, including depression and anxiety; or the biochemical changes resulting from cancer processes. Ask your physician for personalized advice from an oncology-trained dietitian or nutritionist if you're having trouble eating and maintaining your weight. Here we offer some information about how to approach nutrition and exercise after cancer.

Fundamentals for Good Health

The National Cancer Institute (NCI) estimates that at least 35 percent of all cancers are linked to diet. For women, this is as high as one half of all cancers. Good nutrition is vital for a healthy immune system, which protects us and provides us with resistance to cancer. Maintaining a healthy weight is also critical for a healthy immune system and a higher energy level. To maintain a healthy weight, it's important to balance nutrition with physical activity, to lose weight if you are overweight, and to limit alcohol consumption.

Nutrition Guidelines

The foods you choose will make a difference in your health and survivorship. Eating right can help you regain your strength, rebuild tissue, and feel better. Eating right starts with selecting a variety of foods every day, because no one food contains all the nutrients you need. Here are the fundamentals of eating a healthy and varied diet.

- **Focus on plant-based foods.**
  Raw or cooked vegetables, fruits, and fruit juices provide the vitamins, minerals, and fiber you need. Go for color with fruits and vegetables—nature's food rainbow of deep yellow, orange, green, and red.
- **Emphasize whole grains and legumes.**
  Foods like whole-grain tortillas, oats, brown rice, beans, and lentils are good sources of complex carbohydrates, vitamins, minerals, and fiber.
- **Go easy on fat, salt, sugar, alcohol, and smoked or pickled foods.**
  Try lower-fat cooking methods such as broiling, steaming, and poaching rather than frying or charbroiling.
- **Select low-fat milk products and small portions of lean meat, fish, and/or skinless poultry.**
  Eat no more than six to seven ounces per day. The key here is healthy protein, which is also available from vegetable sources such as soy.

The Connection between Dietary Fat and Cancer

Recent studies indicate that many of the hormone-related cancers (breast, colorectal, and prostate) are linked to excess calories and weight, especially central adiposity, known as "belly fat." As Jack LaLanne would say, "Your waist line is your lifeline." Do all you can to reduce your waist to half your height or less, so that you have a minimal amount of this potentially harmful belly fat. When you eat more dietary fiber and less animal fat such as by following a Mediterranean Diet (described later in this chapter), you are eating healthfully not just to reduce your risk of cancer, but also to prevent or manage other chronic conditions such as heart disease or diabetes.

A panel of nutritionists and scientists at the National Institutes of Health (NIH) found that people in the United States eat far too many saturated and animal fats, which are harmful, and not enough beneficial fatty acids. We should adjust our diets to focus on the omega-3 fatty acids found in oily fish (or supplements of fish oil) and some nuts, seeds, and vegetables. In addition, we should also limit our intake of processed foods, animal products, and fried foods filled with omega-6 fatty acids.

When you have cancer, fats or oils from sources that contain more of the beneficial fatty acids are useful to boost calories and support your immunity. Examples of helpful foods include olives (and olive oil), avocados, grapeseed, and nuts (almonds, walnuts, and pistachios). Nuts are particularly good, as are nut butters and seeds (sunflower or pumpkin). Tahini is a paste made from sesame seeds and is another tasty spread or dip.

Eating Tips During Cancer Treatment

Eating well is a vital way to give you that extra edge as you participate in your own recovery. Empower yourself with healthful foods for this important time in your life. Each time you choose a fruit, vegetable, or protein-rich food, you are giving your body what it needs to fight the cancer. Improved nutrition can also help you withstand the side effects of chemotherapy, radiation, and surgery.

Some treatments can make eating difficult or distasteful. Below are specific suggestions to help you with some of the most common treatment-related problems. Even if some of these suggestions are in conflict with the basic high-fiber/low-saturated fat concepts of cancer prevention with which you are familiar, remember that your overriding priority at this time is to maintain a reasonably constant body weight.

For Chewing and Swallowing Difficulties

- Eat soft foods prepared with moist heat (e.g., soups, stews, eggs, pastas, quiches, casseroles).

- Add gravy, sauces, butter, mayonnaise, or salad dressings to make food easier to swallow.
- Avoid highly seasoned, spicy, tart, or acidic foods (no citrus fruits, tomatoes, chilies).
- Avoid alcohol and smoking (this is true for everyone, of course!).
- Consider eating cold foods, which can be soothing if there are sores in the mouth. Just avoid very cold temperatures, and consider using a straw.
- Keep your caloric intake high by using meal replacement drinks (e.g., Ensure®) or try one of the energy-boosting recipes in this book.
- If you have trouble swallowing soups, try using a cup or glass instead of a spoon. Avoid very hot soups.
- Try carbonated drinks, which might be easier to swallow. Allow them to sit at room temperature to reduce carbonation.

For Diarrhea

- Avoid high-fiber foods that contain a great deal of roughage (whole-wheat breads or cereals, raw fruits and vegetables), except for bananas, cooked vegetables with seeds or skins, dried beans and nuts, and popcorn. Cucumber and lettuce might be difficult to digest.
- Eat water-soluble, fiber-rich foods (applesauce or puree; psyllium or Metamucil®).
- Don't drink with your meals, but drink plenty of water in-between meals. Hydration is very important. Fatigue is often an early sign of dehydration. Use rehydration beverages where appropriate, such as Powerade® or Pedialyte®.
- Eat frequent, small, snack-type meals, rather than three large ones.
- The food and liquids you eat and drink should be warm or at room temperature, rather than very hot or ice cold.
- For severe diarrhea, restrict your diet to clear, warm liquids such as broth, flat ginger ale, tea, or apple juice for one day. Check with your doctor if diarrhea persists more than one day.

For Nausea and/or Vomiting

- Eat and drink slowly.
- Eat small, frequent meals.

- Avoid greasy, fatty, and fried foods.
- Rest after meals.
- For nausea early in the morning or before a meal, try a cracker or dry toast.
- Make up for lost calories when you feel more comfortable.
- If cooking odors make you feel nauseated, try microwaving. Use a strong venting fan while you are cooking, or eat outside if the weather permits. Try frozen or chilled foods, as they give off less odor.

For Loss of Appetite

- If you aren't hungry at dinnertime, make breakfast or lunch your main meal. Similarly, if you aren't hungry first thing in the morning, eat more later in the day.
- Eat more frequently but have smaller amounts of food.
- Keep snacks readily available in your purse or in the car.
- Always make food look attractive with garnishes or place settings.
- Experiment with tastes; you might find that things you didn't like before, you like now.
- Try cold or room-temperature foods, which might be more appealing.
- Consider having a glass of wine or beer, which might increase your appetite (check with your doctor first, in case alcohol doesn't mix with a medication).
- Increase the caloric intake of the foods that you do eat with a small amount of "light" (less strongly flavored, not fewer calories) olive oil.
- Try some of the commercially prepared food supplements. Ensure®, Boost®, Benecalorie®, or Polycose® are powdered, unflavored supplements of starch (available from most good pharmacies or drugstores), and add liquid drops to break down the lactose. For diabetics, Glucerna® has a lower glycemic load, which keeps blood sugar more constant. Add fresh berries or juice for variety and additional botanical factors. Try one of the energy-boosting recipes in this book.
- Snack on freeze-dried black raspberries, which are particularly rich in phytonutrients.

Treatment-Related Nutrition Concerns

Traditional chemotherapy and radiation therapy can cause, and might affect, nutrient absorption. There are many products that can be used to supplement reduced food intake, such as high-calorie and/or high-protein ready-to-drink or easily mixed liquid preparations. Some of these are called "elemental," because the nutrients don't require any additional digestion and are readily absorbed even by very sensitive digestive systems. These products can be used along with regular meals, in-between meals, or instead of meals. When you need to get more protein into your diet, try

- protein-fortified beverages with 1/4 to 1/3 cup of nonfat dry milk or whey protein to 1 cup of liquid milk;
- Greek style yogurt;
- tofu, a non-dairy way to add protein to foods (comes in firm and soft textures).

Some people find that treatment with radiation or chemotherapy affects their ability to tolerate simple sugars such as lactose or milk sugar. Typical symptoms include bloating, cramping, or gas several hours after eating milk products. To assist in digesting dairy products, we recommend adding an enzyme such as Lactaid® (available in tablets or liquid drops) to break down the lactose. In addition, using lactose-reduced dairy products might make it possible to use milk and other dairy products, which are an excellent source of calories and protein. Some people also benefit from including a broader type of digestive enzyme such as Wobenzyme-N® or similar product.

Nutrition and Chemotherapy

- Drink plenty of fluids (up to 2 liters total), with most of it coming from clear liquids such as water, apple juice, clear broths, or Jell-O®. Avoid caffeine-containing liquids such as tea, coffee, and colas, as these are dehydrating.
- Eat small frequent amounts of food rather than large meals for easier digestion.
- Eat crackers, Melba toast, pasta, and baked potatoes if you feel nauseated.

- Use the concept of the "Expedient Diet," and make up for eating less healthfully when you have more strength.
- Eat avocado—an excellent source of calories, essential fatty acids, potassium, and glutathione—often unless it is not recommended by your doctor (if on Procarbazine® or other medication requiring a low-tyramine diet).

Dietary advice for a combination regimen advises to avoid fatty foods; eat small quantities of bland flavors; and avoid alcohol, highly spiced foods, or very acidic foods (cranberries, pineapple, lemons, etc.). What you would take home from this is to focus on vegetables; lean meats moistened in liquids, in stews, or in soups; and whole-grain cereals. Many chemotherapy regimens affect your blood cell count. If not contraindicated, a hematinic (blood-building) supplement might be recommended. Always check with your oncologist.

For More Information...

For expert guidance and specifics about how to achieve good nutrition during cancer treatment, see the Web site of Carolyn Katzin, MA, CNS, MNT: www.cancernutrition.com.

Whether I participated in yoga, Mending the Mountains, kayaking, fly fishing, 5K training, cooking classes, or the wide variety of educational activities offered by CSC—the Cancer Support Community has been there for me and others dealing with cancer. I always know that entering the CSC building will provide me with compassion and the emotional support I may need that day. For the CSC staff that 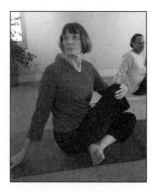 *walked beside me while I negotiated the challenges of my cancer journey, I have the deepest gratitude and appreciation.*

BETH D'ATRI,
community member, Cancer Support Community, Montana

Unexpected Anti-Cancer Foods

- Garlic. Allicin (allythio sulfinic allyl ester) is a weak anti-cancer agent found in garlic. Recognized as early as 1550 BC as a treatment for cancer.
- Milk thistle (Silymarin). This herb might assist in detoxification and general support of the liver detoxification enzyme systems. Useful after chemotherapy.
- Coenzyme Q10. This is another antioxidant that can be beneficial during treatment. Take 50–150 milligrams per day as ubiquinol or as directed by your nutrition professional.
- Green papaya, guava, and pineapple. Many tropical fruits contain natural enzymes that might be beneficial preventively and during treatment.

Natural Energy Drinks

Many treatments for cancer can leave you feeling depleted of energy. Not only that, but food might also taste bland and uninteresting. Here are some recipes to stimulate your appetite and lift your spirits in a natural way. A garnish of fresh fruit or mint adds appeal.

Fruit Shake

1 cup plain low-fat, Greek style yogurt
1 ripe banana
A few drops vanilla extract
1 teaspoon honey
1 teaspoon coconut (optional)

Blend a few ice cubes for a few minutes in a blender, then add the ingredients, and blend until smooth. The banana can be replaced with frozen strawberries, raspberries, half a papaya or mango, or a few chunks of pineapple.

Fruit Juice Smoothie

2 cups apple juice
1 ripe banana
½ cup fresh or frozen strawberries or blueberries
½ cup pineapple juice

Combine ingredients in a blender. Serve chilled.

Energy Drink

Dry Mix
1 cup peeled almonds
1 cup sesame seeds
2 tablespoon protein powder (protein sources are from soy
  isolate [soybeans], whey or casein [milk protein], and/or
  albumin [egg white]).

Combine ingredients in a blender, and blend until fine. This mix can be preserved in the refrigerator for up to two weeks in a sealed jar. When you're ready to use it, blend with chilled fresh mix (below) and drink as a meal enhancer or replacement. Use protein powder alone if other ingredients are not available.

Fresh Mix
1 ripe banana
1 cup fruit juice (apple, cranberry, or similar)
½ cup mineral water
Natural sugar to taste (optional)

Combine ingredients with 1 tablespoon of the dry mix in a blender. Sip slowly. You can also add fresh berries to enhance the taste of canned energy products, like Boost® or Ensure®, etc.

"Immuno-Soup"

This vegetable-based soup is high in immune-building nutrients. It is easily digested and makes a filling meal, despite being low in calories. It's also high in dietary fiber, which is supportive of colon health. A diet consisting of 25 to 30 grams of fiber each day improves the internal regulation of hormones (more than 35 grams of fiber might interfere with mineral metabolism and is not recommended). This recipe makes three to four bowls of this delicious soup.

1 head of celery
1 bunch parsley

½ pound green beans
4 zucchini
1 pound fresh spinach, beet greens, or chard
½ green bell pepper
½ red pepper
1 bunch scallions
1 large potato (Yukon gold are good)
3 medium carrots
½ head cauliflower or 1 head of broccoli
1 turnip or rutabaga
1 parsnip
2 cloves minced fresh garlic
Herbs to taste (thyme, rosemary, oregano, marjoram, etc.) Any
  other vegetables are possible—experiment with seasonal and
  favorite varieties

Wash, slice, chop, or grate all of the vegetables into even-size pieces. Place root vegetables (carrots, potatoes, turnip, rutabaga, or parsnip) into a large pot. Half fill with water and bring to a boil. Cover and simmer for 10 minutes. Add all of the other ingredients, and season to taste. Return to the boil and cook for another 1 to 2 minutes uncovered. Cover and simmer for another 40 minutes. Adjust seasoning, and serve hot or cold. This soup improves with age. Cool rapidly, and keep refrigerated, or freeze serving-sized portions for a quick meal. Make sure you reheat thoroughly, and boil for at least 2 minutes when reheating. There are many anticarcinogenic botanical factors or phytochemicals in vegetables, which help your immune system. This soup is a good way of getting your daily protection of plant-based nutrients. The soup contains less than 3 grams of fat (beneficial type) and 12 grams of protein for under 150 calories. Tamari, soy sauce, or Bragg Liquid Aminos improve the flavoring. You can add more carbohydrate energy by adding brown rice, barley, noodles, canned beans, or corn. Serve with hot bread.

The Mediterranean Heart-Healthy Diet

The Mediterranean Diet is one of the easiest diets to adopt and maintain on a long-term basis because it does not require radical restriction of total amounts of fat or carbohydrate. Calorie intake should be appropriate for maintaining a normal body weight. Guidelines include:

- Eat an abundance of natural, whole plant foods, including vegetables, fruits, and salads. Eat some at every meal and aim for nine or ten servings daily (one small fruit, 1/2 cup of chopped vegetables, or 1 cup of raw vegetables). Often, this means adding just one or two more servings each day.
- Include whole-grain, high-fiber breads and whole-grain pasta in your meals and snacks.
- Keep saturated fat to a minimum: choose chicken, lean cuts of red meat, and nonfat dairy products, and use butter and cheese in moderation.
- Incorporate fatty fish in your diet, especially salmon, sardines, herrings, trout, and tuna. These are good sources of omega-3 fatty acids. Vary the type of fish.
- Use olive oil as a source of monounsaturated fat. Include avocado often.
- Eat frequent servings of peas, beans, legumes, and nuts. Include small quantities (eight to ten) of almonds, walnuts, pecans, and other tree nuts often.
- Drink low to moderate amounts of alcohol. Wine, especially red wine, is a good choice. Consumption should be limited to one drink daily for women, two drinks daily for men.

Avoid the following:

- Foods high in sugar. Restrict to less than 15 grams per serving.
- Trans-fatty acids, which are found in processed foods labeled as containing "partially hydrogenated" oil. Avoid labels containing more than 3 grams of saturated fat per serving.
- Processed "starchy" carbohydrates, such as food made with white flour (e.g., bagels).
- Oils high in omega-6 fatty acids, such as corn, sunflower,

safflower, soybean, or peanut oil. This is contrary to some of the earlier heart-healthy advice given. Further information now shows that the ratio of omega-6 to omega-3 fatty acids is very important and should be reduced by restricting omega-6 fatty acid rich foods, and increasing omega-3 fatty acid rich foods (salmon, flaxseed). A simple way to improve this is to look for omega-3 fortified foods, where the docosahexaenoic acid (DHA) or eicosapentaenoic acid (EPA) is derived from algal sources so they don't taste fishy.

Digestive Enzymes Explained

Digestive enzymes are proteins that assist in the breakdown of food components such as proteins, carbohydrates, and fats. Smaller fragments of food are more digestible or can be absorbed into the body from the intestinal tract. Many people find that supplements of enzymes assist during chemotherapy, possibly helping to induce programmed cell death, or apoptosis.

Life today is so stressful that most of us don't secrete sufficient digestive enzymes. This results in intestinal discomfort and gas. Supplemental digestive enzymes can be helpful in reducing these symptoms, making you more comfortable during your cancer treatment. In fresh foods, the enzyme Bromelain is found in fresh pineapple, and the enzyme papain is in fresh papaya.

Exercise and Physical Activity

Exercise is the performance of physical activity that requires you to use energy. To keep your muscles functioning as well as possible, it's important to exercise as much as your condition allows. Exercise helps prevent problems that are associated with immobility, such as stiff joints, breathing problems, constipation, skin sores, poor appetite, and mental changes.

It's not unusual to lose strength and become deconditioned as a result of cancer treatments, regardless of your previous level of fitness. Fatigue, pain, and the emotional adjustments that might accompany major changes in your body resulting from cancer treatment—such as being too weak to perform activities of daily living without assistance—can also take a toll. Many people have found that participating in some form of exercise helps them gradually increase their endurance and ability to function more independently, and this can have emotional benefits as well.

Customize your exercise to match your level of energy and ability. Start with small steps until you build strength to do more: take a walk every day, and incorporate active or passive range-of-motion exercises as instructed by your nurse, doctor, or physical therapist. It's not in your best interest to stay on the couch with little movement or to let others do for you what you can manage yourself. Start with just five to ten minutes each day and work your way up to the recommended thirty or more minutes per day. Low-impact activities, such as yoga and T'ai chi, can help to focus the mind, alleviate tension and anxiety, reduce stress, and provide you with a renewed sense of wholeness and well-being.

Some people might benefit from physical rehabilitation services that are designed to help you function as normally as possible. These services are carried out by physical and occupational therapists and rehabilitation counselors under the direction of a physician in the hospital, an outpatient setting, or your own home. Physical therapy can help you to regain strength following major surgery; occupational therapy can help increase the strength and coordination of your body or to reevaluate your ability to return to your daily activities; and rehabilitation counseling can help you deal with the emotional impact of your disability.

In doing physical exercise, remember not to confuse "active" with "overactive." You need rest and relaxation during and after cancer treatments. Exhaustion can weaken physical and emotional defenses, and fatigue can make you feel depressed and discouraged.

Exercise: It's No Joke

Even a little exercise goes a long way, and it has proven benefits. Exercise

- keeps or improves physical abilities;
- aids with sleep;
- lowers feelings of anxiety and depression;
- reduces impact from side effects such as nausea and fatigue;
- reduces "chemo-brain" (better clarity with learning and thinking);
- improves blood flow and lowers the risk of blood clots;
- improves balance, and lowers the risk of falls or broken bones;
- lowers the risk of heart disease and osteoporosis;

- aids with weight control;
- improves self-esteem;
- improves sexual functioning.

Taking the Best Care of Yourself

Because cancer treatment and fighting the disease can take all of your energy and then some, maintaining your health and wellness throughout treatment and recovery is essential. Attention to your diet and exercise priorities can not only make you feel better, but also potentially ward off recurrence. It's absolutely critical that you monitor your diet, get lots of rest, and exercise as often as you can to keep your body and soul at their optimum cancer-fighting best.

Patient Action Plan

- **Make good nutrition and exercise a priority in your life.**
  Though they sound hard, nutrition and exercise are the best steps you can take for yourself. Aim to eat a plant-based diet with healthy fats and more whole grains, and exercise at least a few minutes every day—ideally thirty minutes or more each day.
- **Manage side effects with dietary changes.**
  Consider ways to recover from the side effects of cancer treatment with the nutrition tips outlined in this chapter.
- **Consider the help of a dietitian with a specialty in cancer care.**
  Because each person's nutritional needs are very individual, you should see a nutritionist or dietitian to assist you in making healthful food choices.
- **Customize your exercise plan until you regain strength to do more.**
  If exercise is difficult because you are tired, weak, or in pain, customize your exercise plan to help you rebuild your strength, sleep better, and ultimately reduce discomfort (but don't avoid exercise).
- **Good nutrition and exercise offer powerful benefits.**
  Don't underestimate the benefits of diet and exercise on your life now and into the future.

Chapter 16

Facing the Road Ahead Together
Survivorship

I have made many wonderful friends, and I have lost many courageous friends. I feel a sense of purpose when I'm able to help other cancer patients navigate through the rough waters of a cancer diagnosis... my life has more meaning.

ALI DESIDERIO,
community member, Cancer Support Community, San Francisco Bay Area

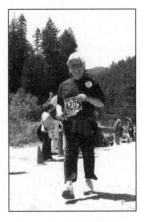

HE TERM "CANCER SURVIVOR" has different meanings for each person. Being a survivor can refer to anyone diagnosed with cancer from the time of diagnosis through the rest of his or her life. The Centers for Disease Control and Prevention actually considers survivors to be anyone affected by the diagnosis of cancer, including family members, friends, and caregivers. You might not personally relate to the term "survivor"—maybe "warrior" is more your speed, or nothing at all—but many use the term to describe those who take an active and positive role in their own future.

Survivorship is complex. For a person who has completed cancer treatment, it can include feelings of relief, pride, and compassion about life and wellness; feelings of abandonment when frequent medical visits are no longer required; and fear of the unknown—wondering if the cancer will return. For many survivors, cancer has to be managed like a chronic illness, which means thinking about cancer for many years after treatment is complete with follow-up care and possibly recurrent cycles of disease, treatment, and recovery. Survivorship involves medicine, mind, and body. It includes being able to manage life with an understanding that the future is unknown for all of us. We can control our well-being, and we can remind ourselves that every day and every moment right now can be special.

A Prescription for Survivorship

After treatment ends, many people go home without an understanding of what's next. As a short- or long-term survivor, you need to be the primary person in control of your own health. However, the coordination of follow-up care for survivors across a range of health professionals is a well-documented problem in our current health care system. Also, not all doctors take the time to help patients plan for all that is needed after treatment is done. The result can be inadequate follow-up care and poorer health outcomes.

Unfortunately, in a recent Cancer Support Community (CSC) research project called MAPP (Mind Affects the Physical), 90 percent of those who responded (758 of 844) did not receive a Survivorship Care Plan (SCP), while 96 percent said that they would have liked one (*Wall Street Journal*, October 11, 2011). The good news is, in the past several years, oncologists, patients and advocates have stepped up and are pushing for a "survivorship prescription" for every person diagnosed with cancer. Here we share a successful survivorship care plan strategy offered by the Institute of Medicine (IOM).

> *At first, cancer was a bad word—but eventually, it becomes just another word. Take the capital "C" off and you're not afraid of it.*
>
> ALFREDO DELAGARTA,
> *community member, Cancer Support Community, Greater Miami*

Wall Street Journal Reports...

Some patients who had treatments years ago are encountering delayed side effects such as heart problems, nerve damage, osteoporosis, and secondary cancers. Nearly 90% of respondents said they had at least one physical, psychological, or social

problem that was moderate to severe.
("The New Front in Breast Cancer: After Treatment Ends." The
Wall Street Journal: Health Journal. October 11, 2011)

Survivorship Care Planning—A Call To Action!

Survivors deserve quality health care for as long as it is needed. When cancer treatment is done, work with your doctor to develop an SCP. This is a plan for wellness that can help ensure that you continue to receive the best health care possible. It includes important information about your medical experiences to be shared with your current and future health care team members. SPCs are intended to ensure that long-term care is addressed for each individual. They are designed to ensure clear communication between you and your care providers, especially if you move, change jobs or insurers, or even doctors. Be sure to keep a copy of your plan, and to also give a copy to each of your doctors.

Although there is no single standard, the IOM recommends that an SPC include five elements, including

- A treatment summary, including diagnosis, test and results, tumor characteristics and types, details of treatment (initiation/completion dates), and treatment side effects;
- the timing and content of follow-up visits;
- tips on maintaining a healthy lifestyle and preventing recurrent or new cancers;
- legal rights affecting employment and insurance;
- availability of psychological and support services.

"Patients completing primary treatment should be provided with a comprehensive care summary and follow-up plan that is clearly and effectively explained. This 'Survivorship Care Plan' should be written by the principal provider(s) who coordinated oncology treatment."

(Institute of Medicine, From Cancer Patient to Cancer Survivor: Lost in Transition, *p. 151)*

Great Resources for Survivors

- LIVESTRONG (www.livestrong.org; "care plan").
The site includes a wide variety of information for survivors.
The purpose is to provide a starting point for you to become
more informed about important matters that might be
affecting your life as a survivor and to provide ideas about
steps you can take to learn more.
- American Society of Clinical Oncology (www.cancer.net/patient).
The ASCO provides clear information (search "survivorship")
about adjusting to various changes in your life following
cancer treatment and offers information about the Institute of
Medicine report on survivorship.
- Cancer Transitions (www.cancersupportcommunity.org).
The program provides information that addresses four
core issues for successful survivorship: exercise, nutrition,
emotional and social issues, and medical management.
- Facing Forward: Life after Cancer Treatment (www.cancer.net).
A program by the National Cancer Institute created to share
common feelings and reactions that many people have after
treatment ends. It also offers some practical tips to help
survivors through this time.

Coping with Changes

Even though friends and family members might suggest that
you "forget about it," each person must seek individual ways of
coping with whatever uncertainties and insecurities he or she
has in being a cancer survivor. Here are a few suggestions for you
from other cancer survivors.

- Get emotional, spiritual, and practical help if you need it,
regardless of how long treatment has been over. Support
groups, psychotherapy, educational workshops, rides to the
hospital, spiritual counseling, etc., are all normal needs of
people with cancer.
- Find out about medications and mechanical aids to treat or
reduce disability or discomfort, such as decreased mobility,

sexual dysfunction, and other physical limitations.
- Learn from others who have the same problems—join a support group, go to a class, and/or connect with someone who has had similar surgery or other treatments.

If Cancer Returns

The fear of cancer recurring and health-related worries ("Is this just a headache, or has the cancer spread?") are the most persistent anxieties associated with cancer survivorship. These fears are often greatest just before an upcoming follow-up visit or annual checkup. The challenge is to learn to live in the moment and balance the fear of recurrence with the desire to enjoy health and wellness. Research from CSC's Cancer Transitions program has shown that social support, combined with moderate exercise and improved diet, actually helps to decrease health-related worries and improve the quality of life for survivors.

If cancer does return, there's no question that it's upsetting and challenging. Yet there are still things you can do to regain control and manage the fears. Many people cope surprisingly well with recurrences or second cancers because they know what to expect, are more knowledgeable about treatment options, and know how to find support. They have learned to employ "patient-empowerment" strategies that help them retain control and hope in the face of uncertainty. In fact, during this period, many people find support groups or individual counseling to be of greatest value.

"Taking one day at a time" has real value when you are faced with a difficult challenge like recurrence. It's not just an old saying without meaning; it means keeping your mind focused on what you need to get done right now, today. It's important for you and your family to avoid looking for reasons for the recurrence. Despite popular literature to the contrary, there are no guarantees about preventing recurrences of cancer. No matter how much a person diets, prays, seeks treatments, etc., cancer might recur—and no one is to blame.

Survivors of most types of cancer may live with a series of recurrences or in chronic states of illness for many years. Having a constructive attitude and maintaining good communications can help you and those who care for you live as normally as you are all able.

Make Life Better, Not Bitter: Adjusting to Your New Normal

You might be keenly aware that cancer isn't something that's easily forgotten. Worrying about the future isn't the same as planning for your future. Worrying prevents you from living your life now. Try to focus on the things you can control and keep your mind busy with things you can manage in your day-to-day moments. Allow yourself to step away from anxious or bitter feelings that accompany cancer, and allow yourself to enjoy the rest of your life. It's important to stay involved with family, friends, and activities. It's important to focus on the here and now. This is one of the best ways to keep your mind in a positive place—by doing the things that you love.

There can also be long-term side effects from both the cancer and the treatment, that, depending on the type of cancer involved, must be dealt with. These can range from changes in your sexual experiences to physical changes after cancer surgery to ongoing fatigue. Being a survivor involves acknowledging and accepting these losses and changes and learning how to manage them over time with follow-up care, counseling, diet and exercise changes, or other helpful strategies. It also means understanding that there is a "new normal" for your life—and that this "new normal" is not bad—it's just different, and it's something faced not only by you, but by almost all cancer survivors.

Life's Priorities Can Change

Having a potentially life-threatening or long-term disease like cancer often leads people to examine their lives and look for meaning. You might change your life's priorities to

- make time to do things that make you happy;
- spend more positive time with family or friends—or find someone to love;
- seek a more meaningful job or volunteer opportunity;
- focus on your health: quit smoking, eat better, exercise more;
- become more spiritual or seek ways to relax and feel more at peace with yourself;
- inspire those you love to focus on the good things in life;
- seek counseling or join a cancer support group.

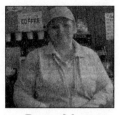

I'm so glad to be done...so grateful to be in remission. Cancer made me a better person....I'm forever changed, [but also] forever grateful for all of the awesome people who have blessed my life, both at the Cancer Support Community and beyond.

BECKY MORGAN,
community member, Cancer Support Community, Greater Lehigh Valley

Finding New Meaning

Having cancer can be challenging at first, but often gives way to a silver lining: You have a chance to look back on your life and all you've been able to accomplish. Though there might be some regrets, most likely there are also many triumphs to celebrate—and many stories to pass on to others in your circle of family and friends.

Perhaps you're reflecting on just how much everyone in your life has meant to you. Or maybe you're honoring them in your own way for what they have become to you as you've traveled this difficult road together since the time of your diagnosis. Whatever's on your mind and in your heart at this moment, you've likely come to the realization that there's no better time than the present to create lasting memories for special people in your life.

In whatever form you choose to express yourself, creating living legacies can be therapeutic for you—and healing for those around you. The best part is, you needn't work on any of these projects alone, unless you choose to do so.

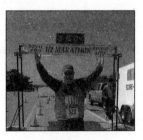

A three-hour Healing through Poetry workshop led me to try writing poetry. Once convinced that I didn't need to know any of the "rules of poetry," I found I liked it [because] it enabled me to release some frustrations that I had buried. So far, I've written about twenty-five poems and continue to write.

DONALD H. WINSLOW,
community member, Cancer Support Community, Delmarva

Create a Living Legacy

You can celebrate your life by

- making a video of special memories;
- reviewing or arranging family photo albums;
- charting or writing down your family's history or family tree;
- keeping a daily journal of your feelings and experiences;
- making a scrapbook;
- writing notes or letters to loved ones and children;
- reading or writing poetry;
- creating artwork, knitting, or making jewelry;
- giving meaningful objects or mementos to loved ones;
- writing down or recording funny or meaningful stories from your past;
- planting a garden;
- making a tape, CD, or playlist of favorite songs;
- gathering favorite recipes into a cookbook.

Source: "Coping with Advanced Cancer," National Cancer Institute, NIH Publication #05-0856

A Circle Journal of Love:

A Story to Honor the Lives of David and Joan Frieder

When David Frieder was diagnosed with cancer, he and his wife, Joan, of Philadelphia, created a journal that made an impact on everyone in their family. At first, the plan was for the children and grandchildren to fill in the pages, but it wasn't long before Joan and David began their entries, "We couldn't help ourselves," Joan said. "We just had to see what everyone was writing in that journal."

The entries were poignant. Joan's daughter Sally once wrote: "You've always shown me how a father can really love his children and how a man can really love his wife. With your guidance, I could never settle for less. You've shown such bravery and character—both you and Mom with this new chapter in your lives. And, as with most things, you will be an example and mentor for us all to learn from, so that we will be better and stronger in the end. You both are my greatest friends. We are all here to help you fight. I love you both."

David appreciated the overriding and powerful message that the circle journal conveyed: His cancer was, in fact, a family disease—and they were all together in the fight for his recovery, no matter where the journey took them.

Facing the Road Ahead

Dr. Harold Benjamin advised patients to "make plans for the future." If you do so, then you're instantly recognizing that there's indeed still plenty of time left in your life. Wherever you may be in your treatment, thinking optimistically about the future is the key to survival. Your doctors and health care professionals are trained experts. By working closely with them on the best treatments available, as well as making plans for the future, however uncertain it might be, you're doing everything you can to get through your cancer experience with peace and dignity. In this way, you'll be the inspiration of all those who know and love you—and that's one very meaningful legacy.

Patient Action Plan

The small things that you do every day to maintain your normal routine will help prepare for the bigger challenges you may have to face in the near or distant future.

- **Create a Survivorship Care Plan with your doctor.**
  Assemble a record of your medical history; summary of your cancer diagnosis and treatment; and follow-up plan for health care.
- **It's okay to feel overwhelmed by the unknown.**
  Perhaps you had your heart set on moving to another city or getting a new job, and now you're wondering if that will ever happen. Plenty of people have proven that dreams don't have to come to an end because of cancer, but the "whens" and "hows" might need to be modified.
- **Keep moving ahead one step at a time.**
  Know that it might take a little longer to achieve everything you want.

- **Know that you're not alone and that there's, indeed, a future that will be rewarding.**
  Of course, you didn't ask for this challenge, but once you're in it, there's always something you can do to make a difference.
- **Create some lasting ways to communicate your feelings.**
  Communicate with your loved ones in the form of art, poetry, scrapbooking, or video.
- **Prepare your will, living will, and advanced directives ahead of time.**
  Many people with cancer find that putting these documents in place relieves them of some anxiety about how their wishes about dying will be honored (see Chapter 10 for more practical considerations).
- **Communicate with your family and your doctor.**
  Be honest about your needs, wishes, and expectations for end-of-life care, including hospice services.
- **Seek out a counselor, spiritual advisor, or support group to explore feelings and concerns.**

Afterword

By Ann Benjamin and Joanna Bull

WE BELIEVE THIS BOOK, *Reclaiming Your Life After Diagnosis: The Cancer Support Community Handbook*, combines much-needed information with the concrete actions that are at the heart of the Cancer Support Community's (CSC's) mission: *To ensure that all people impacted by cancer are empowered by knowledge, strengthened by action, and sustained by community.*

Joanna continues to be actively involved in this remarkable story as it moves on to its next iteration. She engaged in psychosocial support as early as the 1970s, followed by years at The Wellness Community, and then founded Gilda's Club, where "*Living* with cancer, whatever the outcome," was also applied to family and friends in an innovative planned and structured support environment. She sees the merger of Gilda's Club Worldwide with the CSC as, simply, the most direct and effective way at this time to reach still more people who are touched by cancer.

Ann, whose father, Harold Benjamin, founded The Wellness Community and who has grown up in the milieu of his original, brilliant "Patient Active" concept formatted at The Wellness Community, is dedicated to the future of the organization as it continues to serve cancer patients and their families. She has watched, as Harold had hoped, that someday, "The Wellness Community would be put out of business as the cure for cancer was found." Although we continue to passionately hope that this will occur, so many more families are now affected and need the kind of continued support that this merger, the *Cancer Support Community Research and Training Institute*, and this insightful book, *Reclaiming Your Life After Diagnosis*, will bring.

Joanna and Ann, along with CSC under Kim Thiboldeaux's extraordinary and talented command, have combined their inclusive and complementary concepts together to form a basis for the next historic chapter

197

of patient, family, and social-networking support—one that will serve the present day and the changing needs of those living with cancer. This exciting collaboration has given the CSC parent organization the necessary and timely heft to pursue newly defined research collaborations that are leading to still more innovative programs and initiatives. The new Cancer Support Community Research and Training Institute in Philadelphia is certain to continue to break new ground, and this new edition of *Reclaiming Your Life After Diagnosis* will bring those findings to the public at large.

We're proud to continue to be a part of this truly remarkable movement and to have contributed these brief words to this revised and updated edition of what was already an important contribution to the field of psycho-oncology. Its publication marks yet another benchmark in the advancement of support for all people touched by cancer, everywhere.

Acknowledgments

*r*eclaiming Your Life After Diagnosis: The Cancer Support Community Handbook, is a culmination of the history and philosophy of both The Wellness Community and Gilda's Club—now the Cancer Support Community. As we go to press, we celebrate the merger of these two organizations, joining forces and advancing a bold new mission: *To ensure that all people impacted by cancer are empowered by knowledge, strengthened by action, and sustained by community.* We are pleased to share our program philosophy; our lessons learned over the years; some helpful tips; and many enriching stories from our determined, passionate, funny, inspirational community members.

We would like to extend a special thank you to Dr. Mehmet Oz for sharing his insight and wisdom with our community and for dedicating himself to a healthier world. Thank you also to Ann Benjamin and Joanna Bull for their inspiration and unwavering commitment to our work and philosophy.

Next we would like to acknowledge the contributions of the entire Cancer Support Community Headquarters Staff: Ivy Ahmed, MPH, MCHES; Susan Michelson Brown, MSW, MBA; Debbie Rosenberg Bush; Joanne Buzaglo, PhD; Michael Feroz; Sara Goldberger, LCSW-R; Marie Gough; Alexandra Gubin, LGSW, LMSW; Allison Harvey, MPH, CHES; Vicki Kennedy, LCSW; Jay Lockaby, MSS, MLSP; Mark Meinke; our policy advisor Libby Mullin; Christina Raia; Lynn Ryker; Maria Smith, MA; Susan Viana; and Jackie Wieber. You are a top-notch team and it is an honor to work with you. We would particularly like to acknowledge Katina Jones and Erica Weiss, MPH, MSUP, for their dedication, commitment, and tireless work on this project. It was truly a labor of love, and we are profoundly grateful for their efforts. Thank you also to Linda Miller, RN, MSN, OCN; Ashley Varner, MSW, MBA; Supriya Srinivasan, PhD; Margo Michaels, MPH; Barbara Hoffman; and Carolyn Katzin, MS, CNS, MNT, for their important contributions to this text.

Next, we extend a special thank you to all Cancer Support Community affiliate Executive Directors/CEOs, Program Directors, Local Staff, Facilitators, Local and National Board Members, and Local and National Professional Advisory Board Members for your profound support of our mission and for the work you do each and every day to better the lives of all people impacted by cancer.

In addition, we would like to recognize the many corporations, foundations, and individuals who have provided critical financial support to the Cancer Support Community and our affiliate network over the years. Your generosity has made our work possible.

We would also like to thank and acknowledge our friends and colleagues who made this project a reality: Ivan Kronenfeld, Carl Koerner, and Nathalie Casthely from Koerner and Kronenfeld Partners; Frank Weimann and his team at The Literary Group; Glenn Yeffeth and the team at BenBella Books; Ken Kaufman and Matt Fagin at Skadden, Arps, Meagher & Flom LLP; Andy Sandler from BuckleySandler LLP; and, our dear friend and staunch supporter, Holly Page Hoscheit.

Finally, we would like to thank and acknowledge all those people affected by cancer who have attended our programs, both in person and online. You are the true inspiration for this book and you are the force that leads us to do this work each and every day. We hope that the Cancer Support Community, in some small way, has touched you and helped you in your cancer journey.

—Kim Thiboldeaux and Mitch Golant

WOULD LIKE TO THANK my many teachers, mentors, and guides along the way who have taught me always to seek purpose in my work and in my life and to dedicate myself wholly to any task I undertake, no matter how large or small. These include: Susan Cohen Smith, Warren Dennis (in memoriam), Ian Portnoy, Christopher Wolf, Jeff Travers, Frank Condella, Kevin Rigby, Bill Ashbaugh, Harry and April Davidow, Jack Wickens, Ellen Stovall, Chuck Scheper, Jill and Tom Durovsik, Laura Wheat, Diane Perlmutter, and Neil Bassett.

I would also like to thank with all my heart my friends and family who have supported me in every phase of my life and have shown unparalleled excitement about this project. A special thank you to my parents, Bert and Joann, for their love, their dedication to family, and the joy they exude each and every day; and to my siblings (by birth and by marriage), nieces, and nephews for their love and support and commitment to living life in the service of others.

Finally, I would like to thank my coauthor on this project, Mitch Golant. Mitch has been at the Cancer Support Community practically since the beginning. His dedication and compassion are unmatched and his talents beyond measure. Thank you, Mitch, for all that you do for people affected by cancer.

—Kim Thiboldeaux

N APRIL 1985, I began facilitating support groups at The Wellness Community. At that time, we were in a little yellow house in Santa Monica, California, where I had the great good fortune of having Dr. Harold Benjamin, PhD, The Wellness Community's founder, as my mentor, friend, and partner for over twenty years. Today, Dr. Benjamin's seminal idea—the idea of the "Patient Active"—has permeated and positively influenced our understanding of how a patient's attitudes, actions, and beliefs impact the cancer experience. *Reclaiming Your Life After Diagnosis: The Cancer Support Community Handbook* could not have been written without his teachings and dedication to all people with cancer.

I would also like to acknowledge my colleagues and friends throughout the psychosocial oncology field who have supported the Cancer Support Community's growth and progress over the last thirty years. In particular, I am grateful to David Spiegel, MD; Janine Giese-Davis, PhD; Mort Lieberman, PhD; and Andy Winzelberg, PhD, who mentored me in doing research in a community setting. I am also deeply indebted to Stephen Lepore, PhD; Barbara Andersen, PhD; Jeff Belkora, PhD; Margo Michaels, MPH; Deane Wolcott, MD; Jimmie Holland, MD; Matt Loscalzo, MSW; Julia Rowland, PhD; Barry Bultz, PhD; Alan Valentine, MD; and Diana Jeffery, PhD—all of whom are masters in the science of caring. Thank you also to Joel DeGrands and Jeremy Lundberg, for helping the Cancer Support Community implement online support groups and serve cancer patients in innovative ways. In 2008, the Cancer Support Community launched the first community-based Cancer Survivorship Research & Training Institute in Philadelphia, PA. I owe tremendous gratitude to Jill Durovsik, Susan Michelson Brown, Kim Thiboldeaux, the Cancer Support Community Board of Directors and especially Joanne Buzaglo, PhD, for her leadership and passion in translating research into practice that is now reflected in the content of this new book.

To my wife, Susan Golant, who has been my life partner and whose love and enduring support are at the heart of all things good and possible.

Finally, my coauthor, Kim Thiboldeaux, whose tireless energy and belief that great good can come from our joining together in a common purpose are an inspiration and embody true community.

—Mitch Golant

Bibliography

Andersen, B.L., L.M. Thornton, C.L. Shapiro, et al. "Biobehavioral, Immune, and Health Benefits Following Recurrence for Psychological Intervention Participants." *Clinical Cancer Research*. (2010): Vol. 16, no. 12, 3270–3278.

Andersen, B.L., H.C. Yang, W.B. Farrar, et al. "Psychologic Intervention Improves Survival for Breast Cancer Patients: A Randomized Clinical Trial." *Cancer*. (2008): Vol. 113, 3450–3458.

Benjamin, H. *The Wellness Community Guide to Fighting For Recovery from Cancer*. Jeremy P. Tarcher/Penguin, 1994.

Bonadonna, B., A. Moliterni, M. Zambetti, et al. "Thirty Years' Follow Up of Randomized Studies of Adjuvant CMF in Operable Breast Cancer: Cohort Study." BMJ Publishing Group Ltd., January 13, 2005. doi:10.1136/bmj.38314.622095.8F.

Butler, L.D., C. Koopman, E. Neri, et al. "Effects of Supportive-Expressive Therapy on Pain in Women with Metastatic Breast Cancer." *Health Psychology*. (2009): Vol. 28, 579–587.

CancerCare, Inc., in cooperation with the IowaCancer Pain Relief Initiative and the Wisconsin Cancer Pain Initiative. "Bill of Rights for People with Cancer Pain." www.cancercare.org. Accessed on October 1, 2003.

Cassileth, B., and G. Deng. "Complementary and Alternative Therapies for Cancer." *The Oncologist*. (2004): Vol. 9, 80–89.

Cawley, M., and L.M. Benson. "Current Trends in Managing Oral Mucositis." *Clinical Journal of Oncology Nursing*. (2005): Vol. 9, no. 5, 584–592.

Changrani, J., M. Lieberman, M. Golant, P. Rios, J. Damman, and F. Gany. "Online Cancer Support Groups: Experiences with Underserved Immigrant Latinas." *Primary Psychiatry*. October 2008.

Classen, C., L.D. Butler, C. Koopman, et al. "Supportive-Expressive Group Therapy and Distress in Patients with Metastatic Breast Cancer: A Randomized Clinical Intervention Trial." *Archives of General Psychiatry. Journal of American Medical Association* (JAMA). (2001): Vol. 58, 494–501.

Cordova, M.J., J. Giese-Davis, M. Golant, et al. "Breast Cancer as Trauma: Posttraumatic Stress and Posttraumatic Growth." *Journal of Clinical Psychology in Medical Settings*. (2007): Vol. 14, 308–319.

Cordova, M., J. Giese-Davis, M. Golant, et al. "Mood Disturbance in Community Cancer Support Groups: The Role of Emotional Suppression and Fighting Spirit." *Journal of Psychosomatic Research*. (2003): Vol. 55, 461–467.

Davidson, D. "Constipation." *Clinical Journal of Oncology Nursing*. (2006): Vol. 10, no. 1, 112–113.

Derogatis, L.R., M.D. Abeloff, and N. Melisaratos. "Psychological Coping Mechanisms and Survival Time in Metastatic Breast Cancer." *JAMA*. (1979): Vol. 242, 1504–1508.

Eaton, L.H., and J.M. Tipton. "Putting Evidence into Practice: Improving Oncology Patient Outcomes." *Oncology Nursing Society*. Pittsburgh (2009): Vol. 4, no. 8, 253–265.

Eggert, J., ed. S.M. Mahon. "Cancer Basics." *Oncology Nursing Society*. Pittsburgh. (2010b): 35–54.

Ettinger, K., T. Stevens-Thorson, et al. *National Comprehensive Cancer Network Nausea and Vomiting Treatment Guidelines for Patients*. (June 2005): Version III.

Fasciano, K., H. Berman, C. Moore, et al. "When A Parent Has Cancer: A Community-Based Program for School Personnel." *Psycho-Oncology*. (2007): Vol. 16, 158–167.

Fawzy, F.I., N.W. Fawzy, C.S. Hyun, et al. "Malignant Melanoma. Effects of an Early Structured Psychiatric Intervention, Coping, and Affective State on Recurrence and Survival 6 Years Later." *Archives of General Psychiatry*. *JAMA*. (1993): 50: 681–689.

Fortner, B., L. Schwartzberg, K. Tauer, et al. "Impact of Chemotherapy-Induced Neutropenia on Quality of Life: A Prospective Pilot Investigation." *Supportive Care in Cancer*. (2005): Vol. 13, no. 7, 522–528.

Fox, Susannah. "The Social Life of Health Information, 2011." Pew Internet & American Life Project. www.pewinternet.org. 2011.

Giese-Davis, J., K. Collie, E.N. Rancourt, et al. "Decrease in Depression Symptoms Is Associated With Longer Survival in Patients with Metastatic Breast Cancer: A Secondary Analysis." *Journal of Clinical Oncology*. (2011): Vol. 28, 1–8.

Giese-Davis J., S. DiMiceli., S.E. Sephton, and D. Spiegel. "Emotional Expression and Diurnal Cortisol Slope in Women with Metastatic Breast Cancer in Supportive-Expressive Group Therapy." *Biological Psychology*. (2006): Vol. 73, 190–198.

Giese-Davis, J., C. Koopman, L.D. Butler, et al. "Change in Emotion Regulation Strategy for Women with Metastatic Breast Cancer Following Supportive-Expressive Group Therapy." *Journal of Consulting and Clinical Psychology*. (2002): Vol. 70, 916–925.

Giese-Davis, J., C. Kronenwetter, M. Golant, et al. "Qualities of 'Support' in Cancer Support Groups." *Annals of Behavioral Medicine*. (March 1999): Vol. 21, Supplement.

Giese-Davis, J., C. Kronenwetter, M. Golant, et al. "Methods to Illustrate Multi-Faceted Dimensions of Group Therapy and Support." *Journal of Methods in Psychiatric Research* (2010 in review).

Glajchen, M., and R. Magen. "Evaluating Process, Outcome, and Satisfaction in Community-Based Cancer Support Research." *Social Work with Groups*. (1995): Vol. 18, 27–40.

Golant, Mitch. "Managing Cancer Side Effects to Improve Quality of Life." *Cancer Nursing*. (2003): Vol. 26, 37–46.

Golant, M., and S. Golant. *What to Do When Someone You Love is Depressed.* 2nd ed. New York: Henry Holt and Company, 2007.

Golant, M., and K. Thiboldeaux. "The Wellness Community's Integrative Model of Evidence-Based Psychosocial Programs, Services, and Interventions." 2nd ed. New York: Oxford University Press, 2010. *Psycho-Oncology.* 473–478.

Golant, Mitch. "The Launch of the Virtual Wellness Community," *The Los Angeles Psychologist.* (March/April 2003): 5–7.

Golant, M., T. Altman, and C. Martin. "Managing Cancer Side Effects to Improve Quality of Life: A Cancer Psychoeducation Program." *Cancer Nursing.* (February 2003): Vol. 26, 1, 37–46.

Golant, M. "Your Role As a Strengthened Ally." *Coping With Cancer.* (March/April 2002), 16.

Golant, M. "Net Gains? The Wellness Community Explores Internet Support Groups for Women with Breast Cancer." *The Los Angeles Psychologist.* November/December 2001, 16–18.

Goodwin, P.J., M. Leszcz, M. Ennis, et al. "The Effect of Group Psychosocial Support on Survival in Metastatic Breast Cancer." *New England Journal of Medicine.* (2001): Vol. 345, 1719–1726.

Gottlieb, B.H., E. Wachala, ed. "Cancer Support Groups: A Critical Review of Empirical Studies." *Psycho-Oncology.* (2007): Vol. 16, 379–400.

Grant, M., M. Golant, L. Rivera, G. Dean, and H. Benjamin. "Developing a Pain and Fatigue Education Program for Ambulatory Patients with Cancer." *Cancer Practice.* (July–August 2000): Vol. 8, no. 4, 187–194.

Groopman, J. *Anatomy of Hope.* New York: Random House, 2004.

Hawkins, R. and S. Grunberg. "Chemotherapy-Induced Nausea and Vomiting: Challenges and Opportunities for Improved Patient Outcomes." *Clinical Journal of Oncology Nursing.* (2009): Vol. 13, no. 1, 54–65.

Helgeson, V.S., S. Cohen, R. Schulz, and J. Yasko. "Group Support Interventions for Women with Breast Cancer: Who Benefits from What?" *Health Psychology 2000:* Vol. 19, 107–114.

Helgeson, V.S., S. Cohen, R. Schulz, and J. Yasko. "Long-Term Effects of Educational and Peer Discussion Group Interventions on Adjustment to Breast Cancer." *Health Psychology 2001:* Vol. 20, 387–392.

Hesketh, P.J., D. Batchelor, M. Golant, G.L. Lyman, N. Rhodes, and D. Yardley. "Chemotherapy-Induced Alopecia: Psychosocial Impact and Therapeutic Approaches." *Supportive Care in Cancer.* (2004): Vol. 12, no. 8, August, 543–549.

Holland, J.C., B. Andersen, W.S. Breitbart, et al. *National Comprehensive Cancer Network Clinical Practice Guidelines in Oncology: Distress Management.* (Version 1, 2010): www.nccn.org. Accessed January 26, 2010.

Holland, J.C., W.S. Breitbart, P.B. Jacobsen, M.S. Lederberg, M.J. Loscalzo, R. McCorkle, eds. *Psycho-Oncology.* 2nd edition. New York: Oxford University Press, 2010.

Holland, J.C., D. Greenberg, M. Hughes, et al. *Quick Reference for Oncology Clinicians: The Psychiatric and Psychological Dimensions of Cancer Symptom*

Management. American Psychosocial Oncology Society (APOS), Institute for Research & Education (AIRE). IPOS Press, 2006.

Holland, J., and S. Lewis. *The Human Side of Cancer: Living with Hope, Coping with Uncertainty.* HarperCollins Publishers, 2000.

Houts, P.S., A.M. Nezu, C.M. Nezu, J.A. Bucher. *The Prepared Family Caregiver: A Problem-Solving Approach to Family Caregiver Education.* Patient Education Counsel. (1996): Vol. 27, 63–73.

Institute of Medicine (IOM). *Cancer Care for the Whole Patient: Meeting Psychosocial Health Needs.* Washington, D.C.: The National Academies Press, 2007.

Kissane, D.W., B. Grabsch, D.M. Clarke, et al. "Supportive-Expressive Group Therapy for Women with Metastatic Breast Cancer: Survival and Psychosocial Outcome from a Randomized Controlled Trial." *Psycho-Oncology.* (2007): Vol. 16, 277.

Lieberman, M., and M. Golant. "Leader Behaviors as Perceived by Cancer Patients in Professionally-Directed Support Groups and Outcomes." *Group Dynamics, Theory, Research, and Practice.* (2002): 6, no. 4, 267–276.

Lieberman, M., and M. Golant. "Professionally Facilitated Internet Support Groups for Women with Breast Cancer." *International Journal of Group Psychotherapy.* 2003 (In revision).

Lieberman, M., and M. Golant. "Comparisons Between Internet and Face to Face Groups: The Expression of Fear and Anger in Breast Cancer Support Groups." *International Journal of Group Psychotherapy.* 2004.

Lieberman, M., M. Golant, and T. Altman. "Therapeutic Norms and Patient Benefit; Cancer Patients in Professionally-Directed Support Groups." *Group Dynamics, Theory, Research and Practice.* (2004): Vol. 8, no. 4, 265–276.

Lieberman, M., M. Golant, J. Giese-Davis, et al. "Electronic Support Groups for Breast Carcinoma, A Clinical Trial of Effectiveness." *Cancer.* (2003): 920–925.

Lieberman, M., M. Golant, A. Winzelberg, et al. "Comparisons, Professionally-Directed and Self-Directed Internet Groups for Women with Breast Cancer." *International Journal of Self Help and Self Care.* (June, 2004): Vol. 2, no. 3.

Lieberman, M., M. Golant, and A. Winzelberg. "Comparisons Between Internet and Face to Face Groups." *Journal of Psychotherapy.* March 2005.

Lieberman, M., A. Winzelberg, and M. Golant. "Online Support Groups for Parkinson's Disease Patients: A Pilot Study of Effectiveness." *Journal of Social Work and Health Care.* June 2005.

Liess, A., W. Simon, M. Yutsis, J.E. Owen, K.A. Piemme, M. Golant, and J. Giese-Davis. "Detecting Emotional Expression in Face-to-Face and Online Breast Cancer Support Groups." *Journal of Consulting and Clinical Pyschology.* (2008): 76, no. 3, 517–523.

Loscalzo, M., K. Clark, J. Dillehunt, R. Rinehart, R. Strowbridge, and D. Smith. "SupportScreen: A Model for Improving Patient Outcomes." *Journal of the National Comprehensive Cancer Network.* (April 2010): Vol. 8, no. 4, 496–504.

Madden, J., and S. Newton. "Why Am I So Tired All the Time? Understanding Cancer-Related Fatigue." *Clinical Journal of Oncology Nursing.* (2006): Vol. 10, no. 5, 659–661.

Magen, R.H., and M. Glajchen. "Cancer Support Groups: Client Outcome and the Context of Group Process." *Research on Social Work Practice*. (1999): Vol. 5, 541–554.

Marrs, J.A. "Care of Patients with Neutropenia." *Clinical Journal of Oncology Nursing*. (2006): Vol. 10, no. 2, 164–166.

Mock, V. (Chair), A.M. Barsevick, C.P. Escalante, P.O. Hinds, T. O'Connor, B. F. Piper, H.S. Rugo, et al. *National Comprehensive Cancer Network Clinical Practice Guidelines in Oncology, Cancer-Related Fatigue*. (2006): Version 1.

National Cancer Institute. "Taking Time: Support for People with Cancer and the People Who Care About Them." National Institutes of Health. Washington, D.C.: (Revised September 1997): no. 98-2059.

National Institutes of Health. "Alternative Medicine: Expanding Medical Horizons. A Report to the National Institutes of Health on Alternative Medical Systems and Practices in the United States." National Institutes of Health. Washington, D.C. (1994): no. 94-066.

Nezu, A.M., C.M. Nezu, S.H. Felgoise, et al. "Project Genesis: Assessing the Efficacy of Problem-Solving Therapy for Distressed Adult Cancer Patients." *Journal of Consulting Clinical Psychologists*. (2003): Vol. 71, 1036–1048.

Owen, J.E., E.O. Bantum, and M. Golant. "Benefits and Challenges Experienced by Professional Facilitators of Online Support Groups for Cancer Survivors." *Psycho-Oncology*. (February 2009): Vol. 18, no. 2, 144–155.

Owen, J., J. Giese-Davis, et al. "Self-Report and Linguistic Indicators of Emotional Expression as Predictors of Adjustment to Cancer." *Journal of Behavioral Medicine*. (2006): 9061–9068.

Smith, T.J., J. Khatcheressian, G.H. Lyman, et al. "2006 Update of Recommendations for the Use of White Blood Cell Growth Factors: An Evidence-Based Clinical Practice Guideline." *Journal of Clinical Oncology*. (July 1, 2006): Vol. 24, no. 19, 3187–3205.

Spiegel, D., and J.R. Bloom. "Group Therapy and Hypnosis Reduce Metastatic Breast Carcinoma Pain." *Psychosomatic Medicine*. (1983): Vol. 45, 333–339.

Spiegel, D., J.R. Bloom, H.C. Kraemer, and E. Gottheil. "Effect of Psychosocial Treatment on Survival of Patients with Metastatic Breast Cancer." *Lancet*. (1989): Vol. 2, 888–891.

Spiegel, D., J.R. Bloom, and I. Yalom. "Group Support for Patients with Metastatic Cancer: A Randomized Outcome Study." *Archives of General Psychiatry*. The Journal of the American Medical Association. (1981): Vol. 38, 527–533.

Spiegel, D., L.D. Butler, J. Giese-Davis, et al. "Effects of Supportive-Expressive Group Therapy on Survival of Patients with Metastatic Breast Cancer: A Randomized Prospective Trial." *Cancer 2007*. Vol. 110, 1130–1138.

Spiegel, D., L.D. Butler, J. Giese-Davis, et al. "Supportive-Expressive Group Therapy and Distress in Patients with Metastatic Breast Cancer: A Randomized Prospective." *Cancer 2007*. Vol. 110, 1130–1138.

Spiegel, D., C. Classen. *Group Therapy for Cancer Patients: A Research-Based Handbook of Psychosocial Care*. New York: Basic Books, 2000.

Stanton, A.L. "Psychosocial Concerns and Interventions for Cancer Survivors." *Journal of Clinical Oncology*. (2006): Vol. 24, 5132–5137.

Stanton, A.L., P.A. Ganz, J.H. Rowland, B.E. Meyerowitz, J.L. Krupnick, and S.R. Sears. "Promoting Adjustment After Treatment for Cancer." *Cancer 2005*. Vol. 104, 2608–2613.

Terrill, A., J. M. Ruiz, and J.P. Garofalo. "Look on the Bright Side: Do the Benefits of Optimism Depend on the Social Nature of the Stressor?" *Journal of Behavioral Medicine*. (2010): Vol. 33, no. 5, 399–414.

Thiboldeaux, K., and M. Golant. *The Total Cancer Wellness Guide: Reclaiming Your Life After Diagnosis*. Dallas: BenBella Publishing, 2007.

Winzelberg, A., et al. "Evaluation of an Internet Support Group for Women with Breast Cancer." *Cancer*. (2003): Vol. 98, 1164–1173.

Zabora, J., K. Brintzenhofeszoc, B. Curbow, et al. "The Prevalence of Psychological Distress by Cancer Site." *Psycho-Oncology*. (2001): Vol. 10, 19–28.

Zabora, J.R., M.J. Loscalzo, and J. Weber. "Managing Complications in Cancer: Identifying and Responding to the Patient's Perspective." *Seminars in Oncology Nursing*. Elsevier. (2003): Vol. 19 (Suppl 2):1–9.

Other Resources:

- American Cancer Society, Cancer Facts and Figures: www.cancer.org
- National Cancer Institute: www.cancer.gov
- National Center for Complementary and Alternative Medicine: http://nccam.nih.gov

Cancer Care for the Whole Patient

Meeting Psychosocial Health Needs 2007
IOM Report Recommendations

www.iom.edu/Reports/2007/Cancer-Care-for-the-Whole-Patient-Meeting-Psychosocial-Health-Needs.aspx

Cancer care often provides state-of-the-science biomedical treatment, but fails to address the psychological and social (psychosocial) problems associated with the illness. This failure can compromise the effectiveness of health care and thereby adversely affect the health of cancer patients. Psychological and social problems created or exacerbated by cancer—including depression and other emotional problems; lack of information or skills needed to manage the illness; lack of transportation or other resources; and disruptions in work, school, and family life—cause additional suffering, weaken adherence to prescribed treatments, and threaten patients' return to health. A range of services is available to help patients and their families manage the psychosocial aspects of cancer. Indeed, these services collectively have been described as constituting a "wealth of cancer-related community support services."

Today, it is not possible to deliver good-quality cancer care without using existing approaches, tools, and resources to address patients' psychosocial health needs. All patients with cancer and their families should expect and receive cancer care that ensures the provision of appropriate psychosocial health services. This report recommends ten actions that oncology providers, health policy makers, educators, health insurers, health plans, quality oversight organizations, researchers and research sponsors, and consumer advocates should undertake to ensure that this standard is met.

Recommendations for Action

Recommendation 1: The standard of care.

All parties establishing or using standards for the quality of cancer care should adopt the following as a standard:

All cancer care should ensure the provision of appropriate psychosocial health services by

- facilitating effective communication between patients and care providers;
- identifying each patient's psychosocial health needs;
- designing and implementing a plan that
  - links the patient with needed psychosocial services,
  - coordinates biomedical and psychosocial care,
  - engages and supports patients in managing their illness and health; and
- systematically following up on, reevaluating, and adjusting plans.

Recommendation 2: Health care providers.

All cancer care providers should ensure that every cancer patient within their practice receives care that meets the standard for psychosocial health care. The National Cancer Institute should help cancer care providers implement the standard of care by maintaining an up-to-date directory of psychosocial services available at no cost to individuals/ families with cancer.

Recommendation 3: Patient and family education.

Patient education and advocacy organizations should educate patients with cancer and their family caregivers to expect, and request when necessary, cancer care that meets the standard for psychosocial care. These organizations should also continue their work on strengthening the patient side of the patient–provider partnership. The goals should be to enable patients to participate actively in their care by providing tools and training in how to obtain information, make decisions, solve problems, and communicate more effectively with their health care providers.

Recommendation 4: Support for dissemination and uptake.

The National Cancer Institute, the Centers for Medicare & Medicaid Services (CMS), and the Agency for Healthcare Research and Quality (AHRQ) should, individually or collectively, conduct a large-scale demonstration and evaluation of various approaches to the efficient provision of psychosocial health care in accordance with the standard of care. This program should demonstrate how the standard can be implemented in different settings, with different populations, and with varying personnel and organizational arrangements.

Recommendation 5: Support from payers.

Group purchasers of health care coverage and health plans should fully support the evidence-based interventions necessary to deliver effective psychosocial health services.

- Group purchasers should include provisions in their contracts and agreements with health plans that ensure coverage and reimbursement of mechanisms for identifying the psychosocial needs of cancer patients, linking patients with appropriate providers who can meet those needs, and coordinating psychosocial services with patients' biomedical care.
- Group purchasers should review cost-sharing provisions that affect mental health services and revise those that impede cancer patients' access to such services.
- Group purchasers and health plans should ensure that their coverage policies do not impede cancer patients' access to providers with expertise in the treatment of mental health conditions in individuals undergoing complex medical regimens such as those used to treat cancer. Health plans whose networks lack this expertise should reimburse for mental health services provided by out-of-network practitioners with this expertise who meet the plan's quality and other standards (at rates paid to similar providers within the plan's network).
- Group purchasers and health plans should include incentives for the effective delivery of psychosocial care in payment reform programs—such as pay-for-performance and pay-for-reporting initiatives—in which they participate.

Recommendation 6: Quality oversight.

The National Cancer Institute, CMS, and AHRQ should fund research focused on the development of performance measures for psychosocial cancer care. Organizations setting standards for cancer care (e.g., National Comprehensive Cancer Network, American Society of Clinical Oncology, American College of Surgeons' Commission on Cancer, Oncology Nursing Society, American Psychosocial Oncology Society) and other standards-setting organizations (e.g., National Quality Forum, National Committee for Quality Assurance, URAC, Joint Commission) should

- create oversight mechanisms that can be used to measure and report on the quality of ambulatory oncology care (including psychosocial health care);
- incorporate requirements for identifying and responding to psychosocial health care needs into their protocols, policies, and standards;
- develop and use performance measures for psychosocial health care in their quality oversight activities.

Recommendation 7: Workforce competencies.

- Educational accrediting organizations, licensing bodies, and professional societies should examine their standards and licensing and certification criteria with an eye to identifying competencies in delivering psychosocial health care and developing them as fully as possible in accordance with a model that integrates biomedical and psychosocial care.
- Congress and federal agencies should support and fund the establishment of a Workforce Development Collaborative on Psychosocial Care during Chronic Medical Illness. This cross-specialty, multidisciplinary group should comprise educators, consumer and family advocates, and providers of psychosocial and biomedical health services and be charged with identifying, refining, and broadly disseminating to health care educators information about workforce competencies, models, and pre-service curricula relevant to providing psychosocial services to persons with chronic medical illnesses and their families; adapting curricula for continuing education of the existing

workforce using efficient workplace-based learning approaches; drafting and implementing a plan for developing the skills of faculty and other trainers in teaching psychosocial health care using evidence-based teaching strategies; and strengthening the emphasis on psychosocial health care in educational accreditation standards and professional licensing and certification exams by recommending revisions to the relevant oversight organizations.

- Organizations providing research funding should support assessment of the implementation in education, training, and clinical practice of the workforce competencies necessary to provide psychosocial care and their impact on achieving the standard for such care set forth in Recommendation 1.

Recommendation 8: Standardized nomenclature.

To facilitate research on and quality measurement of psychosocial interventions, the National Institutes of Health (NIH) and AHRQ should create and lead an initiative to develop a standardized, transdisciplinary taxonomy and nomenclature for psychosocial health services. This initiative should aim to incorporate this taxonomy and nomenclature into such databases as the National Library of Medicine's Medical Subject Headings (MeSH), PsycINFO, CINAHL (Cumulative Index to Nursing and Allied Health Literature), and EMBASE.

Recommendation 9: Research priorities.

Organizations sponsoring research in oncology care should include the following areas among their funding priorities:

- Further development of reliable, valid, and efficient tools and strategies for use by clinical practices to ensure that all patients with cancer receive care that meets the standard of psychosocial care set forth in Recommendation 1. These tools and strategies should include
  - approaches for improving patient–provider communication and providing decision support to cancer patients;
  - screening instruments that can be used to identify individuals with any of a comprehensive array of psychosocial health problems;

- needs assessment instruments to assist in planning psychosocial services;
- illness and wellness management interventions; and
- approaches for effectively linking patients with services and coordinating care.
- Identification of more effective psychosocial services to treat mental health problems and to assist patients in adopting and maintaining healthy behaviors, such as smoking cessation, exercise, and dietary change. This effort should include
  - identifying populations for whom specific psychosocial services are most effective, and psychosocial services most effective for specific populations; and
  - development of standard outcome measures for assessing the effectiveness of these services.
- Creation and testing of reimbursement arrangements that will promote psychosocial care and reward its best performance.

Research on the use of these tools, strategies, and services should also focus on how best to ensure delivery of appropriate psychosocial services to vulnerable populations, such as those with low literacy, older adults, the socially isolated, and members of cultural minorities.

Recommendation 10: Promoting uptake and monitoring progress.

The National Cancer Institute/NIH should monitor progress toward improved delivery of psychosocial services in cancer care and report its findings on at least a biannual basis to oncology providers, consumer organizations, group purchasers and health plans, quality oversight organizations, and other stakeholders. These findings could be used to inform an evaluation of the impact of this report and each of its recommendations. Monitoring activities should make maximal use of existing data collection tools and activities.

Cancer Support Community Affiliates and Advisors

Cancer Support Community
888-793-9355
www.cancersupportcommunity.org
help@cancersupportcommunity.org

DOMESTIC AFFILIATES

ARIZONA

TWC ARIZONA
Phone: 602-712-1006
www.twccaz.org

CALIFORNIA

CSC PASADENA
Phone: 626-796-1083
www.cscpasadena.org

CSC REDONDO BEACH
Phone: 310-376-3550
www.cancersupportredondobeach.
org

CSC SAN FRANCISCO BAY AREA
Phone: 925-933-0107
www.cancersupportcommunity.net

CSC SANTA MONICA
Phone: 310-314-2555
www.cancersupportcommunity
benjamincenter.org

GC DESERT CITIES
Phone: 760-770-5678
www.gildasclubdesertcities.org

TWC VALLEY/VENTURA
Phone: 805-379-4777
www.wellnesscommunityhope.org

DELAWARE

CSC DELAWARE
Phone: 302-995-2850
www.wellnessdelaware.org

FLORIDA

CSC GREATER MIAMI
Phone: 305-668-5900
www.CancerSupportCommunity
Miami.org

CSC FLORIDA SUNCOAST
Phone: 941-921-5539
www.cancersupportsuncoast.org

GC SOUTH FLORIDA
Phone: 954-763-6776
www.gildasclubsouthflorida.org

GEORGIA

CSC ATLANTA
Phone: 404-843-1880
www.cancersupportcommunity
atlanta.org

ILLINOIS

GC CHICAGO
Phone: 312-464-9900
www.gildasclubchicago.org

INDIANA

CSC CENTRAL INDIANA
Phone: 317-257-1505
www.cancersupportindy.org

IOWA

GC QUAD CITIES
  Phone: 563-326-7504
  www.gildasclubqc.org

KENTUCKY

GC LOUISVILLE
  Phone: 502-583-0075
  www.gildasclublouisville.org

MARYLAND

CSC DELMARVA
  Phone: 410-546-1200
  www.cancersupportcommunity.org/
  delmarva

MICHIGAN

CSC GREATER ANN ARBOR
  Phone: 734-975-2500
  www.cancersupportannarbor.org

GC GRAND RAPIDS
  Phone: 616-453-8300
  www.gildasclubgr.org

GC METRO DETROIT
  Phone: 248-577-0800
  www.gildasclubdetroit.org

MISSOURI

CSC GREATER ST. LOUIS
  Phone: 314-238-2000
  www.cancersupportstl.org

MONTANA

CSC MONTANA
  Phone: 406-582-1600
  www.cancersupportmontana.org

NEW JERSEY

CSC CENTRAL NEW JERSEY
  Phone: 908-658-5400
  www.cancersupportcommunity.org/
  cnj

CSC NORTHERN JERSEY SHORE
  The Diney Goldsmith Center
  Phone: 732-578-9200
  www.cancersupportcommunity.org/
  jerseyshore

GC NORTHERN NEW JERSEY
  Phone: 201-457-1670
  www.gildasclubnnj.org

GC SOUTH JERSEY
  Phone: 609-926-2699
  www.gildasclubsouthjersey.org

NEW YORK

GC NEW YORK CITY
  Phone: 212-647-9700
  www.gildasclubnyc.org

GC ROCHESTER
  Phone: 585-423-9700
  www.gildasclubrochester.org

GC WESTCHESTER
  Phone: 914-644-8844
  www.gildasclubwestchester.org

GC WESTERN NEW YORK
  Phone: 716-332-5900
  www.gildasclubwny.org

OHIO

CSC CENTRAL OHIO
  Phone: 614-791-9510
  www.cancersupportohio.org

CSC GREATER CINCINNATI-
NORTHERN KENTUCKY
  Phone: 513-791-4060
  www.cancersupportcommunity.org/
  cincinnati

PENNSYLVANIA

CSC LEHIGH VALLEY
  Phone: 610-861-7555
  www.CancerSupportGLV.org

CSC PHILADELPHIA
Phone: 215-879-7733
www.cancersupport-phila.org

GC DELAWARE VALLEY
Phone: 215-441-3290
http://gildasclubdelval.org

GC WESTERN PENNSYLVANIA
Phone: 412-338-1919
www.gildasclubwesternpa.org

TENNESSEE

CSC EAST TENNESSEE
Phone: 865-546-4661
www.CancerSupportET.org

GC NASHVILLE
Phone: 615-329-1124
www.gildasclubnashville.org

TEXAS

CSC NORTH TEXAS
Phone: 214-219-8877
www.cancersupporttexas.org

WASHINGTON

GC SEATTLE
Phone: 206-709-1400
www.gildasclubseattle.org

WISCONSIN

GC MADISON
Phone: 608-828-8880
www.gildasclubmadison.org

GC SOUTHEASTERN WISCONSIN
Phone: 414-962-8201
www.gildasclubsewi.org

INTERNATIONAL AFFILIATES

CANADA

GC GREATER TORONTO
Phone: 416-214-9898
www.gildasclubtoronto.org

GC SIMCOE MUSKOKA
(FORMERLY BARRIE, ONTARIO)
Phone: 705-726-5199
www.gildasclubbarrie.org

ISRAEL

TWC TEL AVIV
Phone: 972-3-731-5097
www.twc.org.il

JAPAN

CSC Japan
Phone: 81-3-5545-1805
www.japanwellness.jp

Cancer Support Community
National Board of Directors

Cancer Support Community
Professional Advisory Board

Lidia Schapira, MD
  Assistant Professor of Medicine
  Harvard Medical School
  Massachusetts General Hospital
    Cancer Center
  Boston, MA
Kathryn Schmitz, PhD, MPH
  Senior Scholar, Epidemiology
  Associate Professor of Epidemiology
  University of Pennsylvania
  Perelman School of Medicine
  Philadelphia, PA
Karolynn Siegel, PhD
  Mailman School of Public Health
  Columbia University
  New York, NY
George Sledge, MD
  Professor of Medicine and Pathology
  Indiana University Cancer Center
  Indianapolis, IN
David Spiegel, MD
  Jack, Lulu & Sam Wilson Professor
    School of Medicine, Department

of Psychiatry and Behavioral
  Sciences
Psychosocial Treatment Laboratory
Stanford University School of
  Medicine
Stanford, CA
Alan Valentine, MD
  Deputy Chief of Psychiatry
  University of Texas,
  M.D. Anderson Cancer Center
  Houston, TX
Deane L. Wolcott, MD
  Samuel Oschin Comprehensive
    Cancer Institute
  Los Angeles, CA
Jim Zabora, Sc.D.
  Dean, School of Social Work
  The Catholic University of America
  Washington, D.C.

Support, Information, and Financial Resources

Access Project
617-654-9911
www.accessproject.org
- Tips for managing medical debt

American Brain Tumor Association
800-886-2282
www.abta.org
- Patient Education
- Peer Matching
- Referrals
- Support for people living with cancer and their families and friends

American Cancer Society
800-ACS-2345 (800-227-2345)
www.cancer.org
- Advocacy
- Children's Services
- Culturally Specific Resources
- Financial Assistance
- Housing Assistance
- Medical Information
- Patient Education
- Peer Matching
- Prevention/Detection
- Referrals
- Transportation Assistance
- Support Groups
- Survivorship

American Childhood Cancer Organization
855-858-2226
www.www.acco.org
- Advocacy
- Support Groups
- Patient Education

- Referrals
- Medical Information

American Council on Life Insurers
877-674-4659
www.acli.com
- Offers financial assistance to its member organizations

Academy of Nutrition and Dietetics
www.eatright.org
- Offers scientifically based health and nutrition information

American Hospice Foundation
800-347-1413/202-223-0204
www.americanhospice.org
- Advocacy
- Education and training for health care professionals

American Lung Association
800-LUNG-USA
  (800-586-4872)/202-785-3355
www.lungusa.org
- Advocacy
- Culturally Specific Resources
- Patient Education
- Prevention/Detection
- Support Groups

American Pain Foundation
888-615-PAIN (888-615-7246)
www.painfoundation.org
- Advocacy
- Culturally Specific Resources
- Medical Information
- Patient Education
- Support Groups

American Psychosocial Oncology
Society
866-APOS-4-HELP (866-276-7443)
www.apos-society.org
- Individual Counseling
- Referrals

American Society of Clinical
Oncology
888-651-3038/571-483-1780
www.cancer.net
- Financial Information
- Medical Information
- Medical Referrals
- Patient Education

Angel Flight America
918-749-8992
http://angelflight.com
- Transportation Assistance

Association of Oncology Social Work
215-599-6093
www.aosw.org
- Database (to search for oncology
  social workers)
- Financial Resources

Bladder Cancer Advocacy Network
888-901-2666/301-215-9099
www.bcan.org
- Advocacy
- Patient Education
- Support Groups

BreastCancer.org
www.breastcancer.org
- Medical Information
- Patient Education
- Support Groups

Bright Pink
www.BeBrightPink.org
- Education
- Support

CancerCare
800-813-HOPE (800-813-4673)
www.cancercare.org
- Advocacy
- Support Groups

- Individual Counseling
- Patient Education
- Referrals
- Insurance Information
- Financial Assistance
- Transportation Assistance
- Children's Services
- Survivorship
- Culturally Specific Resources

Cancer Fund of America, Inc. (CFA)
800-578-5284
www.cfoa.org
- Medical Supplies (nutrition
  supplements, lotions, food, toys,
  etc.)

Cancer Hope Network
800-552-4366
www.cancerhopenetwork.org
- Peer Matching
- Individual Counseling
- Referrals

Cancer Information Service
National Cancer Institute
800-4-CANCER (800-422-6237)
www.cancer.gov/aboutnci/cis
- Patient Education
- Medical Information
- Prevention/Detection

Cancer Liaison Program
Office of Special Health Issues
Food and Drug Administration
301-796-8460
www.fda.gov (search "Cancer
  Liaison Program")
- Patient Education
- Referrals

Cancer Legal Resource Center (CLRC)
866-THE-CLRC (866-843-2572)
www.disabilityrightslegalcenter.org
- Legal Information and Resources

Cancer Research and Prevention
Foundation
800-227-2732
http://preventcancer.org

- Advocacy
- Patient Education
- Prevention/Detection
- Culturally Specific Resources

Cancer Support Community
National Headquarters
888-793-9355
www.cancersupportcommunity.org
- Patient Education
- Support Groups
- Individual Counseling
- Referrals
- Medical Information
- Children's Services
- Survivorship
- Culturally Specific Resources

CarePages.com
www.carepages.com
- Free patient blogs and Web sites to connect friends and family during a health challenge

CaringBridge.org
www.caringbridge.org
- Free, personal and private Web sites to connect family and friends during a health challenge

Caring Connections
www.nhpco.org
National Hospice and Palliative Care Organization
800-658-8898
- Patient Education
- Referrals
- Hospice

Centers for Disease Control and Prevention Cancer Information
800-CDC-INFO (800-232-4636)
www.cdc.gov/cancer
- Patient Education
- Referrals

Centers for Medicare and Medicaid Services
800-MEDICARE (800-633-4227)
www.cms.gov
- Insurance Information

Center for Mind-Body Medicine
202-966-7338
www.cmbm.org
- Patient Education
- Referrals
- Medical Information

Children's Cause for Cancer Advocacy
202-336-8374
www.childrenscause.org
- Advocacy
- Patient Education
- Referrals
- Medical Information

Chronic Disease Fund (CDF)
877-968-7233
www.cdfund.org
- Financial Assistance

Clinical Studies Support Center
National Cancer Institute
National Institute of Health Clinical Center
301-496-4345
http://ccr.ncifcrf.gov/trials/default.aspx
- Referrals
- Medical Information

ClinicalTrials.gov
U.S. National Institutes of Health
www.clinicaltrials.gov
- Referrals for clinical trials
- Medical Information

Coalition of Cancer Cooperative Groups
877-520-4457/877-227-8451
www.cancertrialshelp.org
- Patient Education
- Referrals
- Medical Information

Colon Cancer Alliance
877-422-2030
www.ccalliance.org
- Advocacy
- Patient Education
- Peer Matching
- Referrals

Co-Pay Relief Program (CPR)
866-512-3861
www.copays.org
• Financial Assistance

Corporate Angel Network
Westchester County Airport
866-328-1313
www.corpangelnetwork.org
• Transportation Assistance

**Education Network to Advance
Cancer Clinical Trials
(ENACCT)**
240-482-4730
www.enacct.org
• Provides education on cancer
clinical trials

Emergingmed.com
877-601-8601 (to speak with a
clinical trials specialist)
www.emergingmed.com
• Patient education on clinical trials
• Medical Information
• Referrals

**Facing Our Risk of Cancer
EMPOWERED (FORCE)**
866-288-RISK (866-288-7475)
www.facingourrisk.org
• Advocacy
• Information
• Support

Family Caregiver Alliance
800-445-8106
www.caregiver.org
• Advocacy
• Culturally Specific Resources
• Patient Education
• Referrals
• Support Groups

Feeding America
800-771-2303
www.feedingamerica.org
• Local and national food assistance
programs

Fight Colorectal Cancer
877-427-2111
http://fightcolorectalcancer.org
• Advocacy
• Medical Information
• Patient Education
• Referrals

Group Loop
Cancer Support Community
888-793-9355
www.grouploop.org
• Children's Services
• Support Groups

HealthCare.gov
www.healthcare.gov
• Resource for health insurance
information

**Health Resources and Services
Administration (HRSA)**
800-638-0742
www.hrsa.gov/gethealthcare/
affordable/hillburton
• Resource for health care facilities
that provide free or reduced-cost
care

HealthWell Foundation
800-675-8416
http://healthwellfoundation.org/
• Financial Assistance

**Inflammatory Breast Cancer Research
Foundation**
877-STOP-IBC (877-786-7422)
www.ibcresearch.org
• Advocacy
• Culturally Specific Resources
• Patient Education
• Referrals

Intercultural Cancer Council
Baylor College of Medicine
713-798-4617
www.iccnetwork.org
• Advocacy
• Patient Education

International Myeloma Foundation
800-452-2873
http://myeloma.org/Main.action
- Culturally Specific Resources
- Individual Counseling
- Medical Information
- Patient Education
- Peer Matching
- Referrals
- Support Groups

Joe's House
877-JOESHOU (877-563-7468)
www.joeshouse.org
- Resource for lodging near
  treatment centers

Kidney Cancer Association
800-850-9132
www.kidneycancerassociation.org
- Advocacy
- Individual Counseling
- Medical Information
- Patient Education
- Referrals

Kids Konnected
949-582-5443
www.kidskonnected.org
- Children's Services
- Culturally Specific Resources
- Individual Counseling
- Patient Education
- Peer Matching
- Referrals
- Support Groups

Leukemia and Lymphoma Society
800-955-4572
www.lls.org
- Advocacy
- Culturally Specific Resources
- Financial Assistance
- Individual Counseling
- Medical Information
- Patient Education
- Peer Matching
- Referrals
- Support Groups

LIVESTRONG
855-220-7777
www.livestrong.org
- Advocacy
- Culturally Specific Resources
- Medical Information
- Patient Education
- Survivorship

Living Beyond Breast Cancer
888-753-LBBC (5222)
www.lbbc.org
- Culturally Specific Resources
- Individual Counseling
- Patient Eduction
- Peer Matching
- Referrals

Lung Cancer Alliance
800-298-2436
www.lungcanceralliance.org
- Advocacy
- Support Groups
- Individual Counseling
- Peer Matching
- Patient Education
- Referrals
- Medical Information
- Culturally Specific Resources

Lymphoma Research Foundation
800-500-9976
www.lymphoma.org
- Advocacy
- Culturally Specific Resources
- Financial Assistance
- Individual Counseling
- Medical Information
- Patient Education
- Peer Matching
- Referrals
- Transportation Assistance

Melanoma Research Foundation
800-MRF-1290 (800-673-1290)
www.melanoma.org
- Advocacy
- Medical Information
- Patient Education

- Prevention/Detection
- Referrals

Men Against Breast Cancer
866-547-MABC (866-547-6222)
www.menagainstbreastcancer.org
- Culturally Specific Resources
- Patient Education
- Peer Matching
- Referrals

Mesothelioma Information Resource Group
888-802-6376
www.mirg.org
- Medical Informaton
- Patient Education
- Referrals

MetaCancer Foundation, Inc.
www.metacancer.org
- Referrals
- Support Groups

Multiple Myeloma Research Foundation
203-229-0464
www.multiplemyeloma.org
- Advocacy
- Medical Information
- Patient Education
- Referrals
- Support Groups

Mylifeline.org
http://mylifeline.org
- Blogs
- Online Support
- Volunteer Calendars
- Web Sites

National Brain Tumor Society
800-770-8287
www.braintumor.org
- Advocacy
- Culturally Specific Resources
- Medical Information
- Patient Education
- Peer Matching
- Referrals

- Support Groups

National Breast Cancer Coalition
800-622-2838
www.breastcancerdeadline2020.org
- Advocacy
- Patient Education
- Referrals

National Cancer Institute
800-4-CANCER (800-422-6237)
www.cancer.gov or http://
    cancercenters.cancer.gov
- Patient Education
- Culturally Specific Resources
- Medical Information
- Prevention/Detection
- Referrals

National Center for Complementary and Alternative Medicine
National Institutes of Health
888-644-6226
http://nccam.nih.gov
- Advocacy
- Culturally Specific Resources
- Medical Information
- Patient Education
- Referrals

National Cervical Cancer Coalition
800-685-5531
www.nccc-online.org
- Individual Counseling
- Insurance Information
- Patient Education
- Peer Matching
- Referrals
- Survivorship

National Children's Cancer Society
314-241-1600
www.nationalchildrenscancersociety.
    org
- Advocacy
- Children's Services
- Financial Assistance
- Housing Assistance
- Insurance Information

- Patient Education
- Referrals
- Transportation Assistance

National Coalition for Cancer Survivorship (NCSS)
888-650-9127
www.canceradvocacy.org
- Advocacy
- Patient Education
- Referrals
- Insurance Information
- Survivorship
- Culturally Specific Resources

National Energy Assistance Referral (NEAR)
866-674-6327
http://liheap.ncat.org/referral.htm
- Provides information on the Low Income Home Energy Assistance Program

National Hospice and Palliative Care Organization
800-658-8898/703-837-1500
www.nhpco.org
- Advocacy
- Hospice
- Individual Counseling
- Medical Information
- Patient Education
- Referrals

National Lymphedema Network
800-541-3259
www.lymphnet.org
- Advocacy
- Individual Counseling
- Patient Education
- Peer Matching
- Referrals
- Support Groups

National Marrow Donor Program
800-MARROW-2 (800-627-7692)
http://marrow.org/advocacy/
- Advocacy
- Culturally Specific Resources

- Financial Assistance
- Housing Assistance
- Individual Counseling
- Insurance Information
- Patient Education
- Referrals
- Transplant Information
- Transportation Assistance

National Organization for Rare Disorders (NORD)
800-999-6673
http://rarediseases.org
- Medication Assistance

National Ovarian Cancer Coalition
888-OVARIAN (888-682-7426)
www.ovarian.org
- Advocacy
- Culturally Specific Resources
- Patient Education
- Referrals

National Patient Travel Center (NPTC)
800-296-1217
www.patienttravel.org
- Flight assistance for treatment or second opinion

Native American Cancer Research
800-537-8295
www.natamcancer.org
- Culturally Specific Resources
- Patient Education
- Prevention/Detection

NeedyMeds
978-865-4115
www.needymeds.org
- Financial Assistance
- Insurance Information
- Referrals

Nueva Vida
202-223-9100
www.nueva-vida.org
- Advocacy
- Culturally Specific Resources
- Individual Counseling

- Patient Education
- Peer Matching
- Prevention/Detection
- Referrals
- Support Groups

The Office of Minority Health
800-444-6472
http://minorityhealth.hhs.gov
- Culturally Specific Resources
- Referrals

Oncolink
215-349-8895
www.oncolink.com
- Culturally Specific Resources
- Medical Information
- Patient Education
- Referrals

Oncology Nursing Society (ONS)
866-257-4ONS (866-257-4667)
www.ons.org
- Patient Education

Oral Cancer Foundation
949-646-8000
www.oralcancerfoundation.org
- Patient Education
- Prevention/Detection

Ovarian Cancer National Alliance
866-399-6262
www.ovariancancer.org
- Advocacy
- Medical Information
- Patient Education Materials
- Referrals

Pancreatic Cancer Action Network
877-272-6226
www.pancan.org
- Advocacy
- Individual Counseling
- Patient Education
- Peer Matching
- Referrals
- Support Groups

Partnership for Prescription Assistance
888-4PPA-NOW (888-477-2669)
www.pparx.org
- Financial Assistance
- Insurance Information
- Referrals

Patient Access Network Foundation (PANF)
866-316-PANF (866-316-7263)
www.panfoundation.org
- Financial assistance

Patient Advocate Foundation
800-532-5274
www.patientadvocate.org
- Advocacy
- Culturally Specific Resources
- Financial Assistance
- Insurance Information
- Medical Information
- Patient Education
- Referrals

The Patient/Partner Project
866-725-7877
www.thepatientpartnerproject.org
- Patient Education
- Peer Matching

Patient Services, Inc. (PSI)
800-366-7741
https://www.patientservicesinc.org
- Financial Assistance

Planet Cancer
http://myplanet.planetcancer.org/
- Patient Education
- Peer Matching
- Young Adult's Services

Prostate Cancer Foundation
800-757-CURE (800-757-2873)
www.pcf.org
- Advocacy
- Patient Education
- Referrals

The Prostate Net
888-477-6763
www.prostatenet.org
- Advocacy
- Patient Education
- Prevention/Detection

Rosalynn Carter Institute for Caregiving
229-928-1234
www.rci.gsw.edu
- Advocacy
- Caregiver Education

Sisters Network
866-781-1808
www.sistersnetworkinc.org
- Advocacy
- Culturally Specific Resources
- Patient Education on breast cancer
- Prevention/Detection

Skin Cancer Foundation
212-725-5176
www.skincancer.org
- Advocacy
- Culturally Specific Resources
- Medical Information
- Patient Education
- Prevention/Detection
- Referrals

Social Security Administration
800-772-1213
www.socialsecurity.gov
- Financial support information

State Health Insurance Assistance Programs (SHIP)
800-633-4227
www.medicare.gov/contacts
- Resource for health insurance questions— particularly Medicare and Medicaid

Support for People with Oral and Head and Neck Cancer
www.spohnc.org
800-377-0928

- Advocacy
- Medical Information
- Patient Education
- Peer Matching
- Referrals
- Support Groups

Survivorship A to Z
www.survivorshipatoz.org/cancer
- Financial Information
- Legal Information

Susan G. Komen Breast Cancer Foundation
877-GO-KOMEN (877-465-6636)
www.komen.org
- Advocacy
- Culturally Specific Resources
- Individual Counseling
- Patient Education
- Prevention/Detection
- Referrals

Thyroid Cancer Survivor's Association
877-588-7904
www.thyca.org
- Advocacy
- Culturally Specific Resources
- Individual Counseling
- Patient Education
- Peer Matching
- Referrals

Together Rx Access
800-444-4106
www.TogetherRxAccess.com
- Medication Assistance

The Ulman Cancer Fund for Young Adults
888-393-FUND (888-393-3863)
www.ulmanfund.org
- Patient Advocacy
- Patient Educational Materials
- Patient Matching
- Referrals
- Support Groups
- Survivorship

United Way
211 (ext. 27 to speak to a
community resource specialist)
http://liveunited.org
- Financial Assistance
- Resource Support

Uniting Against Lung Cancer
212-627-5500
www.unitingagainstlungcancer.org
- Financial Assistance
- Medical Information
- Patient Education

US TOO International Prostate Cancer Education & Support Network
800-808-7866
www.ustoo.org
- Advocacy
- Culturally Specific Resources
- Individual Counseling
- Medical Information
- Patient Education
- Prevention/Detection
- Referrals
- Support Groups

Vital Options International
818-508-5657
www.vitaloptions.org
- Patient Education
- Referrals
- Support Groups

Y-Me National Breast Cancer Organization
800-221-2141
www.y-me.org
- Advocacy
- Culturally Specific Resources
- Financial Assistance
- Individual Counseling
- Patient Education
- Peer Matching
- Referrals
- Support Groups

Young Survival Coalition (YSC)
877-YSC-1011 (877-972-1011)
www.youngsurvival.org
- Age Specific Resources
- Patient Education
- Referrals
- Support Services

Zero-The Project to End Prostate Cancer
888-245-9455 or 202-463-9455
http://zerocancer.org
- Advocacy
- Patient Education
- Prevention/Detection
- Referrals
- Advocacy

Patient Assistance Programs:

If you do not have prescription medication coverage, have limited prescription insurance, or have a number of prescriptions, you might find you are having difficulty paying for all of them. In these instances, Patient Assistance Programs (PAPs) might be available to help. These are funded by state government, charitable organizations, and pharmaceutical companies. Nearly every pharmaceutical company has a PAP for many of the medications that each particular company makes. These programs provide discounted or free medication to people who qualify. Some PAPs will also facilitate an exception and/or appeal process with your insurance company for coverage of particular medications. Although there are financial criteria to qualify for most if not all of these programs, the criteria can be very generous. If you need help, it's wise to apply. In addition to the programs provided by the drug companies, several nonprofit organizations have developed programs to help patients with the prescription costs including co-pays. For more information, you may want to ask an oncology social worker, patient navigator, or oncology nurse or visit www.cancersupportcommunity.org, where many specific private and charitable programs are listed.

Adjuvant therapy: additional cancer treatment given after the primary treatment to lower the risk that the cancer will come back. Adjuvant therapy might include chemotherapy, radiation therapy, hormone therapy, targeted therapy, or biological therapy.

Aggressive cancer: cancer that is fast growing.

Alopecia: hair loss. Alopecia is almost always temporary; hair grows back when therapy is finished.

Anemia: a shortage of red blood cells. This can cause weakness and fatigue.

Angiogenesis: blood vessel formation. Tumor angiogenesis is the growth of new blood vessels that tumors need to grow. This is caused by the release of chemicals by the tumor.

Anti-EGFR: a form of treatment that uses monoclonal antibodies that target members of the EGFR family in order to stop cell growth signals.

Antiangiogenesis: selectively stopping the process of angiogenesis by cutting the blood supply of tumor cells.

Antibody: a protein made by plasma cells (a type of white blood cell) in response to an antigen (a substance that causes the body to make a specific immune response). Each antibody can bind to only one specific antigen. The purpose of this binding is to help destroy the antigen. Some antibodies destroy antigens directly. Others make it easier for white blood cells to destroy the antigen.

Antigen: any substance that causes the body to make a specific immune response.

Anxiety: feelings of fear, dread, and uneasiness that can occur as a reaction to stress. A person with anxiety might sweat, feel restless and tense, and have a rapid heart beat. Extreme anxiety that happens often over time can be a sign of an anxiety disorder.

Apoptosis: a type of cell death in which a series of molecular steps in a cell leads to its death. This is the body's normal way of getting rid of unneeded or abnormal cells. The process of apoptosis may be blocked in cancer cells. Also called programmed cell death.

Benign: not cancerous. Benign tumors might grow larger but do not spread to other parts of the body. Also called nonmalignant.

Biologic agent: a substance that is made from a living organism or its products and is used in the prevention, diagnosis, or treatment of cancer and other diseases. Biologic agents include antibodies, interleukins, and vaccines. Also called biological agent or biological drug.

Biopsy: surgical removal of a small piece of tissue for evaluation under a microscope.

Bio-therapy: a type of treatment that works with your immune system. Also known as immunotherapy. It can help fight cancer or help control side effects (how your body reacts to the drugs you are taking) from other cancer treatments like chemotherapy.

B-lymphocyte: a type of white blood cell normally involved in the production of antibodies to combat infection.

Bone marrow: the spongy material that is found inside our bones. It contains immature cells called stem cells that develop into three types of cells: red blood cells that deliver oxygen and take away the waste product carbon monoxide, white blood cells that protect from infection, and platelets that help the blood clot.

Bowel perforation: hole in the colon that allows stool to leak out of the colon into surrounding tissue resulting in a serious infection.

Cancer: a term for diseases in which abnormal cells divide without control and can invade nearby tissues. Cancer cells can also spread to other parts of the body through the blood and lymph systems.

Cancer vaccine: a type of vaccine that is usually made from a patient's own tumor cells or from substances taken from tumor cells. A cancer vaccine may help the immune system kill cancer cells. Also called cancer treatment vaccine.

CD20 positive: the presence of a specific antigen found on cell surfaces that helps in the growth and maturation of B-lymphocytes, which help the immune system.

Chemoprevention: the use of drugs, vitamins, or other agents to try to reduce the risk of, or delay the development or recurrence of, cancer.

Chemotherapy ("chemo"): treatment with drugs that kill cancer cells.

Colony Stimulating Factor (CSF): a substance that stimulates the production of blood cells. Colony-stimulating factors include granulocyte colony-stimulating factor (G-CSF), granulocyte-macrophage colony-stimulating factor (GM-CSF), and promegapoietin.

Cytokine: a substance that is made by cells of the immune system. Some cytokines can boost the immune response and others can suppress it. Cytokines can also be made in the laboratory by recombinant DNA technology and used in the treatment of various diseases, including cancer.

Depression: a mental condition marked by ongoing feelings of sadness, despair, loss of energy, and difficulty dealing with normal daily life. Other symptoms of depression include feelings of worthlessness and hopelessness, loss of pleasure in activities, changes in eating or sleeping habits, and thoughts of death or suicide. Depression can affect anyone and can be successfully treated. Depression affects 15–25 percent of cancer patients.

Epidermal Growth Factor Receptors (EGFRs): the protein found on the surface of some cells and to which epidermal growth factor binds, causing the cells to divide. It is found at abnormally high levels on the surface of many types of cancer cells, so these cells might divide excessively in the presence of epidermal growth factor. Also called epidermal growth factor receptor, ErbB1, and HER1.

Familial Adenomatous Polyposis (FAP): an inherited condition in which numerous polyps (growths that protrude from mucous membranes) form on the inside walls of the colon and rectum. It increases the risk of colorectal cancer.

Fatigue: a condition marked by extreme tiredness and inability to function due to lack of energy. Fatigue may be acute or chronic.

First-line treatment: initial treatment used to reduce a cancer. First-line therapy is followed by other treatments, such as chemotherapy, radiation therapy, and hormone therapy to get rid of cancer that remains. Also called induction therapy, primary therapy, and primary treatment.

Fluorescence in situ hybridization (FISH): a laboratory technique used to look at genes or chromosomes in cells and tissues. Pieces of DNA that contain a fluorescent dye are made in the laboratory and added to cells or tissues on a glass slide. When these pieces of DNA bind to specific genes or areas of chromosomes on the slide, they light up when viewed under a microscope with a special light.

Gene therapies: a type of experimental treatment in which foreign genetic material (DNA or RNA) is inserted into a person's cells to prevent or fight disease. Gene therapy is being studied in the treatment of certain types of cancer.

HER1, HER2, HER3, HER4: see Human Epidermal Growth Factor Receptors (EGFR)

Human Epidermal Growth Factor Receptor (hEGFR): receptors found on the surface of both normal cells and cancer cells; members of this family are HER1, HER2, HER3, and HER4. It is found in non-normal levels on some types of cancer cells, including breast and ovarian. Cancer cells removed from the body may be tested for the presence of human epidermal growth factor receptor 2 to help decide the best type of treatment.

Human Genome Project: a project started in 1990 by the National Institutes of Health to identify elements of DNA that lead to an increase in genetic and environmental risk factors for all common diseases.

Immune system: the complex group of organs and cells that defends the body against infections and other diseases.

Immunohistochemistry (IHC): a test done on a tissue sample of a tumor to determine EGFR status (usually for colon cancer).

Immunotherapy: see bio-therapy.

Interferon: a biological response modifier (a substance that can improve the body's natural response to infections and other diseases). Interferons interfere with the division of cancer cells and can slow tumor growth. There are several types of interferons, including interferon-alpha, -beta, and -gamma. The body normally produces these substances. They are also made in the laboratory to treat cancer and other diseases.

Interleukin: a group of natural, hormone-like substances produced by white blood cells in the body that play a central role in the regulation of the immune system.

Intravenous (IV): into or within a vein. Intravenous usually refers to a way of giving a drug or other substance through a needle or tube inserted into a vein.

Lymphocytes: a type of immune cell that is made in the bone marrow and is found in the blood and in lymph tissue. The two main types of lymphocytes are B-lymphocytes and T-lymphocytes. B-lymphocytes make antibodies, and T-lymphocytes help kill tumor cells and help control immune responses. A lymphocyte is a type of white blood cell.

Metastasis: the spread of cancer from one part of the body to another. A tumor formed by cells that have spread is called a "metastatic tumor" or a "metastasis." The metastatic tumor contains cells that are like those in the original (primary) tumor. The plural form of metastasis is metastases.

Monoclonal antibody: a type of protein made in the laboratory that can bind to substances in the body, including tumor cells. There are many kinds of monoclonal antibodies. Each is made to find one substance. Monoclonal antibodies are being used to treat some types of cancer and are being studied in the treatment of other types. They can be used alone or to carry drugs, toxins, or radioactive materials directly to a tumor.

Mutation: any change in the DNA of a cell. Mutations can be harmful, beneficial, or have no effect. Certain mutations can lead to cancer or other diseases.

Neuropathy: a nerve problem that causes pain, numbness, tingling, swelling, or muscle weakness in different parts of the body. It usually begins in the hands or feet and gets worse over time. Neuropathy may be caused by physical injury; infection; toxic substances; disease (such as cancer, diabetes, kidney failure, or malnutrition); or drugs, including anti-cancer drugs. Also called peripheral neuropathy.

Neutropenia: a condition in which there is a lower-than-normal number of neutrophils (a type of white blood cell).

Oncologist: a doctor who specializes in treating cancer. Some oncologists further specialize in chemotherapy ("medical oncologists"), radiotherapy ("radiation oncologists"), or surgery ("surgical oncologists").

Oncology nurse: a nurse who specializes in treating and caring for people who have cancer.

Oncology social worker: an individual who is knowledgeable about cancer and the social and emotional effects of the disease and its treatment. A social worker can provide individual, group, or family counseling; help you navigate the health care system; and help to mobilize valuable resources related to financial, transportation, and home care needs.

"Patient Active": a concept at the core of the Cancer Support Community's program philosophy. It states that, "People with cancer who actively participate in their fight for recovery, along with their health care team, will improve the quality of their lives and may enhance the possibility of recovery."

Pharmacogenomics: the study of how a person's genes affect the way he or she responds to drugs. Pharmacogenomics is being used to learn ahead of time what the best drug or the best dose of a drug will be for a person. Also called pharmacogenetics.

Platelets: a tiny piece of a cell found in the blood that breaks off from a large cell found in the bone marrow. Platelets help wounds heal and prevent bleeding by forming blood clots. Also called thrombocyte.

Prognosis: the likely outcome of a disease; the chance of recovery or recurrence.

Proteomics: the study of the structure and function of proteins, including the way they work and interact with each other inside cells.

Radioimmunotherapy: a type of systemic radiation therapy in which a radioactive substance (a radioisotope) is linked to an antibody that locates and kills tumor cells when injected into the body.

Radiation oncologist: a doctor who specializes in using radiation to treat cancer.

Receptor: a molecule inside or on the surface of a cell that binds to a specific substance and causes a specific physiologic effect in the cell.

Relapse: the return of a disease or the signs and symptoms of a disease after a period of improvement.

Remission: a decrease in or disappearance of signs and symptoms of cancer. In partial remission, some, but not all, signs and symptoms of cancer have disappeared. In complete remission, all signs and symptoms of cancer have disappeared, although cancer still might be in the body.

Stem cell: a cell from which other types of cells develop. For example, blood cells develop from blood-forming stem cells.

Survivorship: the physical, psychosocial, and economic issues of cancer, from diagnosis until the end of life. It focuses on the health and life of a person with cancer beyond the diagnosis and treatment phases. Survivorship includes issues related to the ability to get health care and follow-up treatment, late effects of treatment, second cancers, and quality of life. Family members, friends, and caregivers are also part of the survivorship experience.

Targeted therapies: a type of treatment that uses drugs or other substances, such as monoclonal antibodies, to identify and attack specific cancer cells. Targeted therapy might have fewer side effects than other types of cancer treatments.

T-lymphocyte: a type of white blood cell derived from the thymus (hence T cells) involved in controlling immune reactions. Uncontrolled proliferation of this type of cell gives rise to T cell lymphoma/lymphoma.

Tumor suppressor gene: a type of gene that makes a protein called a tumor suppressor protein that helps control cell growth. Mutations (changes in DNA) in tumor suppressor genes may lead to cancer. Also called antioncogene.

Tyrosine kinase inhibitor: a drug that interferes with cell communication and growth and may prevent tumor growth. Some tyrosine kinase inhibitors are used to treat cancer.

Vascular Endothelial Growth Factor (VEGF): a substance made by cells that stimulates new blood vessel formation.

Personal Information Sheets

Personal Information

Medical Record Number: _____

Insurance Plan/Provider Number: _____

Type of Cancer: _Pheochromacytomas Paragang'_

Stage: _____

Date of Diagnosis: _____

Treatment Received to Date: _____

Your Personal Goals for Treatment: _____

_____

_____

_____

_____

YOUR CANCER TREATMENT TEAM				
Name	Specialty	Office Phone	Emergency Phone	E-mail

D✓

Keith Bible

Quick Reference—Contact Numbers

Doctor _Bible_____

Phone _____ E-mail _____

Doctor _Dr Nigori_____ Surgeon

Phone _____ E-mail _____

Doctor _____

Phone _____ E-mail _____

Nurse _____

Phone _____ E-mail _____

Nurse _____

Phone _____ E-mail _____

Social Worker _____

Phone _____ E-mail _____

Hospital _____

Phone _____ E-mail _____

Ambulance _____

Phone _____ E-mail _____

_____

Pharmacy _____

Phone _____ E-mail _____

Pharmacy _____

Phone _____E-mail _____

Insurance _____

Phone _____E-mail _____

Friend/Family Member_____

Phone _____E-mail _____

Friend/Family Member_____

Phone _____E-mail _____

Support Group _____

Phone _____E-mail _____

Building Your Health Care Team

Include your family or primary care physician, surgeon, medical oncologist, radiation oncologist, chemotherapy nurse, social worker, dietitian, physical therapist, etc. You might find it easier to tape business cards in your journal, so we have given you space to do that.

Your Hospital and Treatment Center Contacts

Name_____

Address_____

_____

_____

Phone & Fax_____

E-mail_____

Specialty_____

Web site_____

Name_____

Address_____

_____

_____

Phone & Fax_____

E-mail_____

Specialty_____

Web site_____

Your Health Care Providers

Include your primary care physician, oncologists, nurses, and social workers.

```
┌─────────────────────────────────────┐
│                                      │
│      Tape business card(s) here      │
│                                      │
│                                      │
│                                      │
│                                      │
└─────────────────────────────────────┘
```

```
┌─────────────────────────────────────┐
│                                      │
│      Tape business card(s) here      │
│                                      │
│                                      │
│                                      │
│                                      │
└─────────────────────────────────────┘
```

Name _____

Address _____

_____

_____

Phone & Fax _____

E-mail _____

Specialty _____

Web site _____

Name_____

Address_____

_____

_____

Phone & Fax_____

E-mail_____

Specialty_____

Web site_____

Name_____

Address_____

_____

_____

Phone & Fax_____

E-mail_____

Specialty_____

Web site_____

Name_____

Address_____

_____

_____

Phone & Fax_____

E-mail_____

Specialty_____

Web site_____

Name _____

Address _____

_____

_____

Phone & Fax _____

E-mail _____

Specialty _____

Web site _____

Name _____

Address _____

_____

_____

Phone & Fax _____

E-mail _____

Specialty _____

Web site _____

Name _____

Address _____

_____

_____

Phone & Fax _____

E-mail _____

Specialty _____

Web site _____

Your Health Insurance

Name _____

Address _____

_____

_____

Phone & Fax _____

E-mail _____

Specialty _____

Web site _____

Your Medicare/Medicaid Plan

Name _____

Address _____

_____

_____

Phone & Fax _____

E-mail _____

Specialty _____

Web site _____

Name _____

Address _____

_____

_____

Phone & Fax _____

E-mail _____

Specialty _____

Web site _____

Your Pharmacy

Name _C.V.S._

Address _N. Alpine Rd_

Loves Park ILL.

Phone & Fax _815-6336666_

E-mail _____

Specialty _____

Web site _____

Name _____

Address _____

_____

_____

Phone & Fax _____

E-mail _____

Specialty _____

Web site _____

Name _____

Address _____

_____

_____

Phone & Fax _____

E-mail _____

· Specialty _____

Web site _____

Outside Agencies and Organizations

Include visiting nurse/home health agencies, support organizations, and transportation services.

Tape business card(s) here

Tape business card(s) here

Name _Cancer Support Community_

Address _____

_____

_____

Phone & Fax _____

E-mail _____

Specialty _____

Web site _www.cancersupportcommunity.org_

Name _____

Address _____

_____

_____

Phone & Fax _____

E-mail _____

Specialty _____

Web site _____

Name _____

Address _____

_____

_____

Phone & Fax _____

E-mail _____

Specialty _____

Web site _____

Name _____

Address _____

_____

_____

Phone & Fax _____

E-mail _____

Specialty _____

Web site _____

Other Important Contacts

Include family and friends, neighbors, work associates, clergy, etc.

Name _____

Address _____

_____

_____

Phone & Fax _____

E-mail _____

Specialty _____

Web site _____

Name _____

Address _____

_____

_____

Phone & Fax _____

E-mail _____

Specialty _____

Web site _____

Name _____

Address _____

_____

_____

Phone & Fax _____

E-mail _____

Specialty _____

Web site _____

Appointment Notes

Date: _____

Location: _____

With: _____

Questions I need to ask:

    1.

    2.

    3.

    4.

Action steps following this appointment:

    1.

    2.

    3.

    4.

Questions I need to ask:

    1.

    2.

    3.

    4.

Action steps following this appointment:

    1.

    2.

    3.

    4.

Appointment Notes

Date: _____

Location: _____

With: _____

Questions I need to ask:

   1.

   2.

   3.

   4.

Action steps following this appointment:

   1.

   2.

   3.

   4.

Questions I need to ask:

   1.

   2.

   3.

   4.

Action steps following this appointment:

   1.

   2.

   3.

   4.

Appointment Notes

Date: _____

Location: _____

With: _____

Questions I need to ask:

    1.

    2.

    3.

    4.

Action steps following this appointment:

    1.

    2.

    3.

    4.

Questions I need to ask:

    1.

    2.

    3.

    4.

Action steps following this appointment:

    1.

    2.

    3.

    4.

Appointment Notes

Date: _____

Location: _____

With: _____

Questions I need to ask:

   1.

   2.

   3.

   4.

Action steps following this appointment:

   1.

   2.

   3.

   4.

Questions I need to ask:

   1.

   2.

   3.

   4.

Action steps following this appointment:

   1.

   2.

   3.

   4.

Appointment Notes

Date: _____

Location: _____

With: _____

Questions I need to ask:

    1.

    2.

    3.

    4.

Action steps following this appointment:

    1.

    2.

    3.

    4.

Questions I need to ask:

    1.

    2.

    3.

    4.

Action steps following this appointment:

    1.

    2.

    3.

    4.

Appointment Notes

Date: _____

Location: _____

With: _____

Questions I need to ask:

1.

2.

3.

4.

Action steps following this appointment:

1.

2.

3.

4.

Questions I need to ask:

1.

2.

3.

4.

Action steps following this appointment:

1.

2.

3.

4.

Your Side Effect Tracking Log

A tool to help you track signs of infection and other treatment side effects during your cancer treatment.

Date/ Time/ Treatment Cycle

Your doctor has planned several cycles of treatment for you, which will take place over a period of weeks to months. You can keep track of your schedule here.

1. Monitor Your Side Effects Every Day

Note any of the following symptoms. The symptoms that are underlined should be reported immediately. It is helpful to write your symptoms down to discuss them in detail with your doctor or nurse at your appointment:

- <u>Chills, sweating, fever</u>
- <u>Cough or sore throat</u>
- <u>Redness, pain, heat, or swelling around skin sores, catheters (port-a-cath, PICC line, etc.), or other wounds</u>
- Nausea or loss of appetite
- Tingling sensation in fingers or toes
- Loose bowel movements/diarrhea
- <u>Shortness of breath or trouble breathing</u>
- Extreme fatigue or tiredness
- Dizziness
- Skin sores
- Numbness or tingling
- Loss of appetite or increase in appetite
- <u>Bruising or bleeding</u>
- Mouth sores, bleeding, or thick mucus
- Confusion, depression, or anxiety
- Nausea or vomiting
- Difficulty staying warm
- Pale skin
- Constipation
- Loss of or change in sex drive
- Pain (tell where)
- Rapid heartbeat

- Change in sleeping pattern
- Other

2. Medical Plan of Action

This should be based upon advice from your oncology team.

3. Personal Plan of Action

Include the steps you will take to resolve the problems you have discussed with your oncology team.

4. Other Solutions

Include any solutions not yet mentioned, including support groups, mind-body techniques, wellness techniques, or complementary medicine that you're interested in or currently use. (Please remember to tell your oncology team about any complementary or alternative medical and diet solutions that you use to ensure that they do not complicate your treatment plan.)

5. Record Your Blood Work Results

At office visits, your nurse might do a complete blood count, measuring the level of your neutrophils (infection-fighting white blood cells), hemoglobin, hematocrit, and platelets. These numbers tell your health care team whether you're at risk for side effects such as infection, fatigue, or bleeding. Write down the numbers your nurse gives you for the counts below:

Date: Date the blood count was taken
ANC: Absolute neutrophil count—measurement of infection-fighting neutrophils
Hgb: Hemoglobin—measurement of the oxygen-carrying component of red blood cells
Plt: Platelets—total number of cells that help stop bleeding
Other: You may want to keep track of tumor markers or other tests that are specific to your cancer type and may be important to you

Date/Time Treatment Cycle	1. Side Effects	2. Medical Plan of Action	3. Personal Plan of Action	4. Other
EXAMPLE Date: <u>July 10</u> Time: <u>4:15pm</u> Cycle: <u>1st Chemo.</u>	1) 100.5°F fever 2) tired	1) immediately call M.D. for fever 2) discuss fatigue at next appointment	1) follow M.D. instructions 2) delegate tasks, find time for more rest	1) try an online support group 2) try a low-impact exercise like yoga
Date: Time: Cycle:				
Date: Time: Cycle:				
Date: Time: Cycle:				
Date: Time: Cycle:				
Date: Time: Cycle:				
Date: Time: Cycle:				

5. Blood Work

Date: ___/___/___

ANC: _____

Hgb: _____

Plt: _____

Other: _____

Date/Time Treatment Cycle	1. Side Effects	2. Medical Plan of Action	3. Personal Plan of Action	4. Other
EXAMPLE Date: <u>July 10</u> Time: <u>4:15pm</u> Cycle: <u>1st Chemo.</u>	1) 100.5°F fever 2) tired	1) immediately call M.D. for fever 2) discuss fatigue at next appointment	1) follow M.D. instructions 2) delegate tasks, find time for more rest	1) try an online support group 2) try a low-impact exercise like yoga
Date: Time: Cycle:				
Date: Time: Cycle:				
Date: Time: Cycle:				
Date: Time: Cycle:				
Date: Time: Cycle:				
Date: Time: Cycle:				

5. Blood Work

Date: __/__/__

ANC: _____

Hgb: _____

Plt: _____

Other: _____

Date/Time Treatment Cycle	1. Side Effects	2. Medical Plan of Action	3. Personal Plan of Action	4. Other
EXAMPLE Date: <u>July 10</u> Time: <u>4:15pm</u> Cycle: <u>1st Chemo.</u>	1) 100.5°F fever 2) tired	1) immediately call M.D. for fever 2) discuss fatigue at next appointment	1) follow M.D. instructions 2) delegate tasks, find time for more rest	1) try an online support group 2) try a low-impact exercise like yoga
Date: Time: Cycle:				
Date: Time: Cycle:				
Date: Time: Cycle:				
Date: Time: Cycle:				
Date: Time: Cycle:				
Date: Time: Cycle:				

5. Blood Work

Date: ___/___/___

ANC: _____

Hgb: _____

Plt: _____

Other: _____

Date/Time Treatment Cycle	1. Side Effects	2. Medical Plan of Action	3. Personal Plan of Action	4. Other
EXAMPLE Date: <u>July 10</u> Time: <u>4:15pm</u> Cycle: <u>1st Chemo.</u>	1) 100.5°F fever 2) tired	1) immediately call M.D. for fever 2) discuss fatigue at next appointment	1) follow M.D. instructions 2) delegate tasks, find time for more rest	1) try an online support group 2) try a low-impact exercise like yoga
Date: Time: Cycle:				
Date: Time: Cycle:				
Date: Time: Cycle:				
Date: Time: Cycle:				
Date: Time: Cycle:				
Date: Time: Cycle:				

5. Blood Work

Date: ___/___/___

ANC: _____

Hgb: _____

Plt: _____

Other: _____

Date/Time Treatment Cycle	1. Side Effects	2. Medical Plan of Action	3. Personal Plan of Action	4. Other
EXAMPLE Date: <u>July 10</u> Time: <u>4:15pm</u> Cycle: <u>1st</u> <u>Chemo.</u>	1) 100.5°F fever 2) tired	1) immediately call M.D. for fever 2) discuss fatigue at next appointment	1) follow M.D. instructions 2) delegate tasks, find time for more rest	1) try an online support group 2) try a low-impact exercise like yoga
Date: Time: Cycle:				
Date: Time: Cycle:				
Date: Time: Cycle:				
Date: Time: Cycle:				
Date: Time: Cycle:				
Date: Time: Cycle:				

5. Blood Work

Date: __/__/__

ANC: _____

Hgb: _____

Plt: _____

Other: _____

Date/Time Treatment Cycle	1. Side Effects	2. Medical Plan of Action	3. Personal Plan of Action	4. Other
EXAMPLE Date: <u>July 10</u> Time: <u>4:15pm</u> Cycle: <u>1st</u> <u>Chemo.</u>	1) 100.5°F fever 2) tired	1) immediately call M.D. for fever 2) discuss fatigue at next appointment	1) follow M.D. instructions 2) delegate tasks, find time for more rest	1) try an online support group 2) try a low-impact exercise like yoga
Date: Time: Cycle:				
Date: Time: Cycle:				
Date: Time: Cycle:				
Date: Time: Cycle:				
Date: Time: Cycle:				
Date: Time: Cycle:				

5. Blood Work

Date: __/__/__

ANC: _____

Hgb: _____

Plt: _____

Other: _____

Personal Thoughts

Day/Date: _____

Time: _____

Personal Notes:

Personal Thoughts

Day/Date: _____

Time: _____

Personal Notes:

Personal Thoughts

Day/Date: _____

Time: _____

Personal Notes:

Personal Thoughts

Day/Date: _____

Time: _____

Personal Notes:

Personal Thoughts

Day/Date: _____

Time: _____

Personal Notes:

Personal Thoughts

Day/Date: _____

Time: _____

Personal Notes:

Index

Bold page numbers are definitions.

A

AACR. *See* American Association for Cancer Research (AACR)
abnormal cells, 8–9, 59, 237–38
"AC" (after cancer), 15
ACA. *See* Affordable Care Act (ACA)
ADA. *See* Americans with Disabilities Act (ADA)
adjuvant therapy, **237**
affirmations, 158–59
Affordable Care Act (ACA), 115
Agency for Healthcare Research and Quality, 213
alcohol-based hand sanitizer, 146
alcoholic beverages
  avoid, 104, 108, 110, 176, 179
  limit consumption of, 174, 183
alopecia (hair loss), 48, 53–54, 108–9, **237**
American Association for Cancer Research (AACR), 39
American College of Surgeons, 132, 214
American Council on Life Insurers, 120
American Dietetic Association, 86
American Society of Clinical Oncology (ASCO), 39, 132, 190, 214, 226
American Society of Hematology (ASH), 39
Americans with Disabilities Act (ADA), 120
amino acids, 82
Anatomy of an Illness as Perceived by the Patient (Cousins), 21
The Anatomy of Hope (Groopman), 140
Andersen, Barbara, 139, 164
anemia, 94, 102–4, **237**
anger, 15, 22, 131, 136–37, 139–40
angiogenesis, 59, **237**
annual checkup, 191
antiangiogenesis, 59, **237**
antibody, 57–59, **237**, 241
anti-cancer drugs, 58–59, 240
anti-EGFR, **237**
antigen, 57, 64, **237**, 238

antinausea medication, 99
anxiety, 18, 54, 173, **237**
apoptosis, 11–12, 56, 184, **237**
appetite loss, 106, 110, 177, 180, 184, 261
appointment notes, 255–60
appointment times, 29–30
art therapy, 77
ASCO. *See* American Society of Clinical Oncology (ASCO)
ASH. *See* American Society of Hematology (ASH)
Aspirin, 61
Avastin® (bevacizumab), 59
Ayurvedic medicine, 79, 82

B

"BC" (before cancer), 15
belly fat, 174–75
benign tumors, 8, **237**
Benjamin, Ann, 197–98
Benjamin, Harold, 7, 20–21, 24–25, 195
Bibliographic Information on Dietary Supplements, 87
Bill of Rights for People with Cancer Pain, 99–100
biochemical changes, 173
bioelectromagnetic-based therapies, 84
biofeedback, 77, 99
biofield therapies, 83
biological agent, **237**
biologically based therapies, 79, 81–82
biomarkers, 55, 59, 64
biomarker screening, 55
biopsy, 37, 50–51, **238**
bio-therapy, **238**
blaming yourself, 23–24
blood cancer, 7
blood-clots, 104–5, 110, 185
blood tests, 7, 22, 104
B-lymphocyte, **238**, 240
board certification, 41
body image problems, 133

275

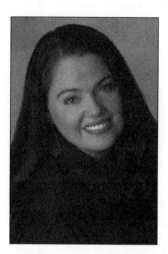

KIM THIBOLDEAUX is President and CEO for the Cancer Support Community (CSC). Kim Thiboldeaux joined The Wellness Community in 2000 as President and CEO. In 2009, the headquarters of The Wellness Community and Gilda's Club joined forces to become the Cancer Support Community, one of the largest providers of social and emotional support worldwide, where Kim has maintained her role as President and CEO. The combined organization is also likely the largest nonprofit employer of psychosocial oncology mental health professionals, advancing the idea that psychosocial care is as important as medical care in the face of a cancer diagnosis. The Cancer Support Community provides social and emotional support through a network of nearly 50 local affiliates, more than 100 satellite locations, and online at www.cancersupportcommunity. org. The organization also maintains a Research & Training Institute in Philadelphia, PA.

Formerly the Director of Patient Relations for Oncology & Transplant at Hoffmann-LaRoche, Inc., Kim brings to this position a wealth of experience in health care, patient education, and national patient advocacy. Kim serves in numerous leadership roles in the cancer and health care communities including: founding board member of ENACCT (Education Network to Advance Cancer Clinical Trials), member of the American College of Surgeons Commission on Cancer, Co-Chair of the Alliance for Quality Psychosocial Care, and Advocacy Board Member of the Ruesch Center for the Cure of GI Cancers at Lombardi Comprehensive Cancer Center. Prior to joining Roche, she served as the Director of Corporate Relations at Whitman-Walker Clinic, a Washington, D.C.-based clinic that provides comprehensive services to people with HIV and AIDS.

Kim co-authored *The Total Cancer Wellness Guide*, which was published by BenBella Books on June 1, 2007. This timely book is a roadmap for all people affected by cancer and offers helpful tips on treatment decisions, side-effect management, social and emotional issues and more. She is also the host of *Frankly Speaking About Cancer with the Cancer Support Community*, an award-winning Internet talk radio show that airs weekly on voiceamerica.com and is aimed at informing and inspiring listeners to live well with cancer.

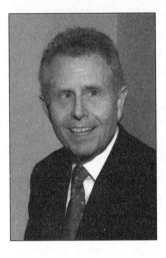

MITCH GOLANT, PhD is a health psychologist and Senior VP of Research & Training for the Cancer Support Community. He has traveled throughout the world introducing CSC's Patient Active Concept to international thought-leaders and psychosocial oncologists. He has been with CSC for over 28 years where he supervised and trained CSC's professional clinical staff. He has facilitated over 6,000 support groups for people with cancer and trained over 400 professionals nationally and internationally in CSC's Patient Active Support Group model. Dr. Golant is widely recognized as a pioneer in the use of information technology in cancer education and support through the delivery of online support groups. He was central to the launch of the award-winning Cancer Support Community Online in both English and Spanish and, as well as Group Loop: Teens. Talk. Cancer. Online. He has presented globally on CSC's Patient Active programs and evidence-based research. He has previously served on the Board of Directors for the American Psychosocial Oncology Society. He received the Los Angeles County Psychological Association's Distinguished Contribution in Psychology Award in October 2011. He is the contributing editor to the *Essentials of Psychosocial Oncology Handbook* (2006) and *The Psychiatric and Psychological Dimensions of Pediatric Cancer Symptom Management* (2008). He is also the co-author of seven books including The Total Cancer Wellness Guide: *Reclaiming Your Life After Diagnosis* (BenBella 2007), *What To Do When Someone You Love is Depressed* (Holt—updated and expanded 2007), and a contributing author of *Psycho-Oncology, 2nd Edition* (Oxford University Press 2010).